About the author
Christine Durham PhD

Christine, educator by training and profession, acquired brain injury as the result of a car accident in 1991. Author of *Doing Up Buttons* (Penguin Books, 1997), and *Chasing Ideas* (Finch Publishing, 2002, translated into Chinese, Korean and Arabic) she has also contributed to the books *Coping for Capable Kids* (Hawker Brownlow Education, 1993) and *Teaching Strategies that Promote Thinking* (McGraw Hill, 2006). Principal of the business 'Talk About Change' she presents to a wide range of audiences. She was invited to compile a presentation for Henry Stewart Talks (UK) for the Biomedical and Life Sciences Collection, and is currently developing a Brain Injury Learning Resource and a book to help children understand brain injury. A mother of four and grandmother of seven, Christine lives with her husband Ted in Melbourne. She was presented with the BrainLink 'Woman of Achievement Award' for 2012 and is the Victorian Senior Australian of the Year for 2014.

Unlocking
my
Brain

Through the labyrinth of Acquired Brain Injury

Dr CHRISTINE DURHAM

JCP
JANE CURRY PUBLISHING

Unlocking my Brain
Through the labyrinth of Acquired Brain Injury
Written by Dr. Christine Durham

First published in 2014 by Jane Curry Publishing

Sections of this book were previously published by Penguin Australia under the title *Doing up Buttons* 1997

PO Box 780, Edgecliff, NSW 2027
AUSTRALIA
www.storyworkspublishing.com
www.janecurrypublishing.com.au

Copyright © Christine Durham 2014

All rights reserved. No part of this book may be reproduced or transmitted in any form or by any means, electronic or mechanical, including photocopying, recording or by any other information storage or retrieval system, without prior permission in writing from the publisher.

National Library of Australia cataloguing-in-publication data:

Author: Christine Durham
Title: *Unlocking my Brain; Through the labyrinth of Acquired Brain Injury*

ISBN 978-1-922190-83-3 (Print edition)
ISBN 978-1-922190-84-0 (Epub Edition)
ISBN 978-1-922190-85-7 (Epdf/Mobi Edition)

Cover and internal images: Shutterstock/istock/Getty Images

Cover and internal design: Deborah Parry
Editorial: Sarah Plant
Production: Jasmine Standfield
Printed in Australia by McPherson's Printing Group

Dedication

To Peter who helped me live

PASSING BY
*Peter thank you for giving me a second chance with life.
Thank goodness it was you who happened to be passing by.
My St George. You saved me from death, or a fate worse than death.
Your cool clear head was the most valiant of swords.
Now I can watch my kids grow up, I can watch my grand kids grow,
And my husband and I can grow wise and old together.*

and
to my family Ted, Helen, Ann, Ken, Rob, Greg,
Tony, Gabrielle,
Alexander, Hannah, Leroy, Lucinda, Spencer,
Sebastian and Ruben
for their love and encouragement.

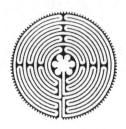

Contents

	Author's note	9
	Introduction	11
1.	The day my life changed	15
2.	I find myself in the labyrinth: Intensive care	19
3.	Ward woes	23
4.	In a room of my own	31
5.	Home among the gum trees	36
6.	Spitting chips!	45
7.	Stuck in a glass box	48
8.	Out of my glass box and into the world	53
9.	Rehab: Trapped in a different labyrinth	55
10.	The more you do the more you see your problems	63
11.	Getaway to the coast	69
12.	University: Trying to find 'Me' and get out of the labyrinth	73
13.	School: Trying to find 'Me' and get out of the labyrinth	77
14.	Reality and unreality clash	86

15.	End of the year my life changed	89
16.	Caught in court — a labyrinth within a labyrinth	93
17.	As time goes by	104
18.	Life goes on!	112
19.	Examining the heart	117
20.	Facing the music	123
21.	Mum and Dad	128
22.	The year of the dove	134
23.	Killing three birds with one stone	138
24.	Getting out of the labyrinth through writing, speaking and listening to others with brain injury	145
25.	Acquiring Better Insight into the Acquired Brain Injury experience	156
26.	Keys to the ABI Cage	169
27.	Issues that locked people in the ABI Cage	172
28.	Things that released people from the ABI Cage	183
	Further Reading	192
	Index	200

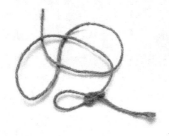

Author's note

One morning, when I was about six years old, my mother was walking me to the front gate to farewell me as I went to school, when we were dismayed to notice that one of the row of standard rose bushes that lined our driveway had fallen over in the wind.

So we went in search of string to reattach it to the support. There was no string in the kitchen drawer, no string in the garage and no string in the garden shed, so Mum took a stocking off the clothes line and used that to retie the rose bush.

That afternoon, walking home from the bus stop, I noticed a piece of string lying in the gutter so I picked it up and proudly presented it to Mum who overacted her delight at this gesture. And so, at the age of six, I became convinced that the thing my mother liked best in the whole world was string! Consequently I discovered and collected bits of string in all sorts of unlikely places, poking out of the sand at the beach, caught on fences and even jammed in a tree. Eventually the back shed was festooned with string. Finding pieces of string taught me an important life lesson: I could find what I was looking for!

This book is an account of my two decade long search, not for string, but for understanding. It tells how I've tried to grapple with, and make sense of, the 'new me' the person I'd become after my life was changed by acquired brain injury (ABI). It is also about searching for happiness. For years after my accident I was tackling so many problems that I felt sure that I would never ever be happy again. However, I've discovered that for me happiness is not getting rid of all my problems, but rather it's about finding out how to accept and cope with them.

I hope that this story can be a string for you, a guide to help you negotiate your own challenging labyrinth.

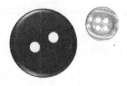

Introduction

We were going out for the first time in many months. I'd almost managed to dress myself — I was so proud. What a surprise for the family! I wanted to wear the antique pearl necklace Ted had bought in Paris. I'd been wearing it when I had the accident. Ann was about to fasten it when she noticed that there was a drop of dried blood on one of the pearls. After she cleaned the pearl she fastened the clasp for me and I turned round to be admired. Ann clucked 'Come here Mum and I'll fix your buttons. You can't go out like that!'

My tiny bubble of self-satisfaction popped. Oh, to be able to do up my own buttons properly! Over the coming months, buttons became a symbol of all sorts of things — small things we take for granted until they disappear — independence, the kindness of my family, being in charge of my life. They stood for putting things together, for size and colour, for skill. My lips and limbs felt as if they were buttoned up. I wanted to unbutton them! But most of all I wanted to button up my life, I wanted to put it together again.

Buttoning up my life involved a journey of self-discovery, from deepest despair at the emotional devastation of brain injury to understanding and emotional growth. The trigger and the outcome of this journey was and is hope.

Since my car accident in 1991 I have been trying to piece together the whole picture of what happened, its ramifications and what I should do to recapture myself. People say to be forearmed is forewarned. I was not. There were no warnings of the obstacles and barriers that lay ahead.

My book *Doing Up Buttons* was published by Penguin Books in 1997. I hoped that by telling my story I could help people who had suffered brain injury to understand some of the issues so they could discuss their feelings and thoughts with their loved ones. I also wanted to give their family, friends and professionals working in the field of brain injury a picture of the personal issues involved in this complex and complicated condition. I was amazed at the contact from readers who said that the book had struck a chord with them. In sharing my personal experience — from being unable to walk, talk, see or think properly through to how I regained my life and found my feet, thoughts and confidence — I had unknowingly voiced the thoughts and experiences of many of the one in 45 people in the community struggling with brain injury.

Readers expressed how the book had encouraged and helped them understand brain injury, loss and change:

'*...so confirming of my head injury*'

'*I take heart from your example*'

'*...it is as though I was looking in a glass at myself and your feelings were mine*'

'*I realised it would give me insights. What I did not expect was the degree of inspiration and encouragement I found.*'

After the book was published I was invited to speak to hundreds of people with brain injury, and to present to a wide variety of audiences in Australia and overseas including leading community organisations, leadership and rehabilitation groups, health professionals and universities. My husband Ted and I formed a speaking business 'Talk About Change'. As well as presenting to groups I was also privileged to listen to stories of people with brain injury. I learnt how they felt 'lost', but that *Doing Up Buttons* had helped them understand they were not alone.

I became even more curious about the brain injury experience and 15 years after my accident, at the age of 63, I embarked on a PhD. This time I was not looking for string, but for factors that negatively and positively affect the lives of people with brain injury. I was in a unique position because I could really understand the problems and people with brain injury were comfortable talking to me. Using symbols and objects I triggered conversations which encouraged people with brain injury and the people who cared for them, to open up and share their brain injury experiences. I've incorporated some of the most important lessons I discovered in the final chapters of this book.

My daughter Helen once gave me a card with picture of a sweet little pig leaping out over some water. Her words were: 'For the woman who, whilst she can't make pigs fly, can get them leaping pretty far (and there's not much difference!)'. Perhaps 'Pigs can leap!' should be the title of this book!

I hope that *Unlocking My Brain* will help people find a way to unlock their brains so they can find a path through their labyrinth.

This story has one aim — to encourage. Remember pigs can leap!

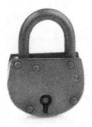

1.
The day my life changed

Two more sums on the board,
Two sums more, two more seconds
And I'd be OK for sure.

I smiled as I straightened up the postcard on the display board in my classroom. I was feeling on top of the world. The postcard fitted perfectly into a space among the colourful posters, pictures and clippings I'd put up for our unit on 'Around the world in 60 days'. It seemed unbelievable that I had written it from so far away only three weeks ago.

> MAY 1991
> My Dear Amigos, hot greetings from Mexico! How are you all? I hope you had great holidays! Mexico is amazing! My conference was amazing! The way I was mobbed by people from all over the world when I read my paper was amazing! The gold and ornate churches are amazing! The ancient ruins are amazing! See! Don't forget to use different adjectives! Ted and I are about to rattle through the dry jungle to Uxmal to climb this massive pyramid. Just as well you broke me in at Wilson's Prom. Camp. Fondest love to you all...
>
> Chris Durham

What experiences and adventures my husband Ted and I had the day I wrote that postcard! I fondly thought of the evening of that day, when we had swum in the teardrop-shaped pool as the sun set in a blaze of crimson and a thousand swallows fluttered down to drink the reflected pink water we were bathing in. What a way to celebrate our silver anniversary — in the land of silver beneath a silver fingernail of moon.

I'd had my paper accepted at a philosophy conference at the university in Mexico City. The atmosphere was exciting, so many people from around the world united in the common belief that the world would be a better place if children were taught to wonder and think. The trip had been a delight; delivering my paper in the vast hall and its reception by people from Iceland to Brazil, the night when the vice-chancellor gave a party in the courtyard of his home, the crazy taxi ride across the city, the deep blue of the sky, the glorious moon and the heart-rending surprise as a Mariachi band burst through the kitchen door. Our Mexican friends had clutched our arms, explaining the words of each song, then the hat was passed round for pesos for the band to play again.

For a decade I had been searching for 'string', for the magic ingredient that, when added to the school curriculum, could enrich and extend the student's thinking. Like a quest for the Holy Grail my journey of discovery had taken me in many directions. I had studied education and curriculum, and was embarking on my Master's degree to try to find something 'special' that would help my students. I believed that philosophy might be the golden substance that would enrich our discussions, making them more powerful and empowering. When I learnt that the next International Philosophy for Children conference was to be held in Mexico I was thrilled. I submitted a paper and, to my delight, it was accepted. Mum and Dad had made travel a vital part of their life and spoke fondly of the elegance, beauty and fascination of Mexico.

I glanced round my classroom as I shut the door. What a busy day it had been. It was good to adventure in far-off places but oh, so good to be safely home. I smiled as I remembered an interview I'd had with the new school principal earlier in the year. We were asked to reveal something about ourselves and I had gathered up some symbols to tell her about my four children. A torn-off strip of white sheet represented Helen, our eldest. She'd worn the ribbon tied around her arm that summer's day when we'd met for lunch at university; apparently it was a protest against the Gulf War. Always working for causes, at 24 she was completing honours in law at Melbourne University. For 22-year-old Ann I'd taken a beautiful piece of silk that she had hand painted. She had just completed a BA in fashion, and was painting, designing, sewing and creating. Ken, who was 20, was represented by a spoon and a book—what a fantastic cook he was! What a pleasure to have about the house, so handy and helpful. He was working on his Arts degree and was slightly obsessed with politics. A music note on a slip of paper represented talented, musical, 15-year-old Rob. I'd missed his company in the car today — he had to catch the train home from school because I had university.

I thought of my 28 school kids. It was wonderful to be back at school. I taught Year Six at Ivanhoe Girls' Grammar, where I'd been for the past 11 years. I found teaching fulfilling and exciting. I completed filling the blackboard with fractions for tomorrow's maths lesson. 'We'll finish this unit tomorrow if it kills me!' I thought.

I tossed the bag containing my reports and papers I'd written for my Master's project on the back seat of the car. It was a calm and pleasant afternoon with the sun breaking through the clouds. I had a busy and interesting evening ahead: first to Melbourne University where I had an aesthetics lecture, then a bite to eat before my Philosophy for Children committee meeting. As I drove to university, a sensation of peace and safety washed over me. Although the trains were on strike the traffic was light; there would be time for a coffee. The traffic lights ahead turned red.

There was no other car on my side of the road. It was eerie, like the calm before the storm. Then I heard and felt a bang.

Blackness. Flashes of bright, piercing, white light, pain, strange sounds of clattering metal, choking, blackness, floating, agony, hell.

Where was I?

What was happening?

A voice floated faintly from far away, 'Is it all right for us to cut off your clothes?' Cold scissors on flesh. Blackness and yet more blackness.

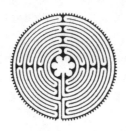

2.
I find myself in the labyrinth: Intensive care

To think I made the news, stopped the traffic, was dramatically rescued, cut out of a car, rode in an ambulance...and I didn't know a thing.

I felt as if I was down a long dark tunnel, being dragged towards what I thought was golden daylight at the end. Then I was out in the blinding sunshine, dazzled by the light. It seemed as if welcoming figures were approaching me. Time stood still. I felt myself move towards them, but suddenly found myself being sucked back along the tunnel, bitterly disappointed. I emerged hovering near the ceiling, looking down at my still body and the people frantically doing things to it. I was in intensive care. The room was dark but I was lit by a pool of brilliant white light. People were all about me. They seemed to be panicking. I felt calm. Calm and detached. I hovered above my tormented body: I could sense that it was me and I could feel the agony. I was watching from the ceiling as several doctors and nurses worked on my body. Later I was aware I was back on the bed with someone insisting, 'You must make a greater effort to breathe or we'll have to insert a tube into your lungs and you won't like that!'

I don't exactly like *this*! Nothing could be worse than this! I must be dreaming!

This is not happening to *me*, a voice inside my head said. More blackness. Words came from afar out of the darkness: 'You've been clipped. You've had a car accident, you're in intensive care in hospital.'

There were painful, yet vague, sensations of being manhandled by different people; each indistinct person had yet another unexpected way to torture me. I was apart yet somehow connected to the weird ceremonies around me. I was central to this hostile act, yet unknowing, mute. I was propped up, lain down, my blood taken, tubes were inserted into my body. At one stage I found myself in the arms of a nurse who was trying to force me to cough and breathe. I had contracted pneumonia and my lung was deflated, I had multiple breaks to over half my ribs.

Sensations of floating through the blackness alternated with sensations of being nailed to my bed, of steel spikes penetrating my body. Each of my keepers fiddled and adjusted the tubes. A tube fell out, blood gushed from the fountain in my wrist. An unseen hand squeezed firmly on the wound to stem the flow. Pain spun up my arm, but I had no words to protest.

Yet another pain surfaced: my tongue. (I'd bitten off a chunk when I had an epileptic fit in the car when I was imprisoned). But again, I had no words to explain so I kept poking out my tongue, grunting and tried to point to it. It seemed ages before someone noticed and painted it with something soothing.

Six days after the accident I had brief flashes of opening my eyes. What crazy world was I in? Spirals of smoke or fog danced around my prone body. Through a hole in the fog I could just see a strange person with two heads. I closed my eyes in disbelief, yet, when I opened them again a similar vision would meet my gaze. Time to retreat into the black world in my mind.

I tried to speak to explain this. Thoughts were in my head but they refused to come out of my mouth.

My mind was locked up. My brain and body were completely detached from each other. My brain was bolted shut, yet somewhere in the depths of my being I had the epiphany that my brain was dependent upon my body and my body was really important to keep my brain alive. My return from the light at the end of the tunnel had also involved another epiphany; I came back from 'the light' with a vivid 'understanding' that the most important thing we own are our own thoughts. Weeks later I reflected that this revelation meant that the secret of me recapturing my life was 'thinking'. My purpose was clear — I had to struggle to keep my body alive so that my brain could discover the secret of thinking!

But I was locked inside this brain and body that could not communicate. It was terrifying. From somewhere came the gestures, noises to explain about the two-headed monsters that inhabited this horrific world. After some time, a white patch of gauze materialised from the shadows to be fixed across my eye with sticky tape. Blessed relief.

According to Helen, during my first few days in hospital members of my family constantly visited, but I was very unresponsive. As I began to realise where I was, I became extremely distressed and overwhelmed by the pain I was experiencing.

I can't remember how the hours passed. About all I can remember was Ted giving me a teaspoon full of jelly and the enormous difficulty I had trying to swallow it. My mouth wouldn't work for talking or eating — was it because of my swollen tongue? Fog continued to dance about me, changing partners with blackness or blinding white light. The music was unearthly metal clanking, moans and the hiss of machines. Frequently a stranger would emerge from the gloom, crank up my bed until I was in a sitting position and take X-ray photos of me. So many that I'm amazed I don't glow in the dark!

On the seventh day I was told I was being transferred out of the dark, quiet dungeon of intensive care to a general ward.

Irrational thoughts like 'Will my family ever find me again?', 'Who is controlling me?', 'Why?', 'Why am I here?', 'Why do I have all this pain?' swirled in my head.

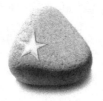

3.
Ward woes

The pain is as if electric drills are ripping bone and nerves.
Can't you turn off the power and silence the drill?

I couldn't see, think or communicate properly. Perhaps someone did try to explain what had happened and was happening to me, but I could not comprehend. All I knew was I was in horrific pain and this was because I had been in a car accident. I had neither thoughts nor words to wonder how or why. I didn't know who I was, or what day it was.

My bed was moved through a labyrinth of endless cream passages, like a giant monster from a movie, bumping and clanging with the attached oxygen bottle, drips, monitors, catheter bag and so on. With each movement it felt as if spikes were being driven into my body. The pain of being transferred into a bed in the new ward caused me to nearly black out. I was relieved to be stationary again. Faint optimism surfaced: 'Now it would be a bit better'. But the torturer's rack had followed me. The pain was still there, along with the noise, confusion and chattering people.

My injuries included closed head injury with diplopia and post-traumatic amnesia; multiple fractures of ribs 1 to 10 on my right with right pneumothorax (the abnormal pressure of air between the lung and the wall of the chest that results in a collapsed lung); multiple fractures of ribs 2 to 5 on the left; fractured right clavicle; fracture of the orbit to my left eye; weakness of right arm and shoulder girdle due to a brachial plexus injury and probable traction on cervical nerve roots; whiplash-type injury to cervical spine; soft tissue injury to thoraco-lumbar discs; and associated ligamentous structures at multiple levels and central vestibular disturbance. In other words I felt crook!

Ted came to see me in the evening. He tried, yet again, to explain that I had been in a car accident: my car had been hit on the passenger side by a person running a stop sign. I was in a chest ward because of my punctured, deflated lung and the pneumonia that had tried to take me down the tunnel to the 'other place' when I was in intensive care.

I lay with the oxygen mask fizzing (what a relief it was when I could have tubes instead of the suffocating mask), a catheter and a forest of tubes going into my neck to monitor my heart and for pain control. The six-bed chest ward did not bring peace. The long night hours were filled with the snores of the man in the bed opposite. At visiting time I had heard his wife say that he was the worst snorer in the world — I could certainly believe that! My bed curtains provided me with some privacy but no sound protection.

The pain in my ribs and back took my breath away, it was like lying on a pile of red-hot spikes, the slightest cough or movement slid another deep spike into my back.

My damaged brain had finally registered that I was gravely ill. Maybe it is from stories from my childhood, but I knew that when you were very ill you had all your hair cut off 'to preserve your strength'. I managed to get through to Helen that I wanted my hair chopped off. At the time I was unable to even lift my head off the pillow but somehow the visiting hairdresser managed to cut my hair by turning my head on the pillow. I didn't feel any stronger but I'd be less trouble now.

The ward was a very noisy place. Besides all the televisions competing in volume with each other, there was the chatter of visitors, doctors' rounds and the nurses' monitoring. I asked to have the curtains drawn about my bed, but every second nurse would pull them back and I didn't have the words to request politely that they be kept shut. The light pierced my un-patched eye.

I can't remember eating, and when the drip was removed I don't think I ate for some time. I had difficulty swallowing and I'd choke. I couldn't taste anything and with both hands feeble I couldn't feed myself. Neither could I explain what was wrong.

My family visited; Ted on his way to and from work. It was a comfort to have him with me but I felt such a nuisance — he always appeared so hassled, so edgy. I felt guilty for causing him extra worry when he was already going through a stressful time of reorganisation at work.

When the children visited, Helen would massage my clenched left hand or my feet; Ann would softly pat my paralysed right hand; Ken would put his strong hand on my leg; and Rob would look shocked and bewildered. Greg, Helen's boyfriend, sat and read to me short stories by Roald Dahl. I couldn't understand what anyone was saying so little did I realise that as he approached the end of each tale he would invent a plausible 'tame' ending to the story because he did not want to upset me.

The saddest visitors were my dear elderly parents who, at that time, were 75 and 78. They would make the hour-long journey daily, negotiating parking and a long walk to the ward to visit me. Looking like two distressed birds, they would search in vain for some slight improvement. Even though I was unaware of much that was going on I could feel their fear and sense the hopeless situation I was in. I could also feel their love. They so desperately needed to cling to something.

Mum would murmur over and over 'My poor broken doll! My poor broken doll!'

I felt all of their dread and despair, but I had nothing to offer, no hope, no polite words. I felt a failure. I couldn't fulfil their expectations. They tried so hard to cheer me up but I could not talk when I had no words, nothing to say that would relieve their suffering. I was also very concerned about Dad driving the long distance to the hospital.

One afternoon Mum remarked, 'What a pretty nightie'. Looking back I realise she was only trying to find something pleasant to say but inside my head roared the thought, 'I don't care about my damned nightie! I can't see, I'm in agony, I don't know who I am, I can't speak properly, I've lost my career, my world has collapsed — life is awful.'

I'm ashamed to say I told Ted to tell them not to come. I just couldn't cope with their sad, unrealistic belief that things would one day be 'normal' or their need to cling to some form of hope. I had no patience or energy to pretend I was even a little better. This was perhaps the most selfish thing I'd ever done. I hated myself but deep down I realised that in order to survive I did not have the energy to comfort them.

Dear friends, colleagues from school, past pupils and their mothers popped in for brief visits. It required a superhuman effort to greet them and make appropriate noises to thank them for gifts and flowers.

I was slowly going mad. The constant noise of televisions and radios, the ever-present nurses, physios, cleaners, visitors and the nurses' insistence on pulling away my curtains of privacy left me at screaming pitch. For hours I would make an 'Arrrr' sound to myself — it made me feel like I was doing something, and it reminded me that I must still be alive.

Ken brought in a tape player so I could listen to some of my favourite music. The music evoked feelings in me about how life had been in the past and tears would roll down my cheeks and drip off my chin. Ken persisted and brought in taped stories. He chose Tolkien's *Lord of the Rings*. Words are inadequate to describe the effect this had on me, the sensation of it all happening in my head. The goblins and warriors, surreal landscapes and strange happenings were all so like the horrific larger-than-life technicolour 3D nightmares and daydreams I was experiencing. I tried to persevere, but it soon became apparent that listening to the radio, music and stories was too disturbing.

I tried reading books and magazines. It was weird trying to do so with all the double images, and I had trouble finding the right word and making sense of what I was reading.

The family tried to keep me interested in happenings at home. Rob had a fancy dress dance at school and Ann found time from running the house to make him an Edward Scissorhands outfit. Rob was brought in to let me see the outfit on his way to the dance. I tried to pretend I was interested in Ann's amazing work but I felt isolated, cut off in my own world of pain. Helen skipped lectures to sit with me. She would rub and massage my hand and chat. Ken also missed lectures to sit with me. I needed them, but I couldn't help feeling I was wrecking their lives.

Although I was on oxygen, I had to have my lungs artificially expanded every couple of hours. This meant having tight straps forced over my head to hold on the mask, an excruciatingly painful sensation when my neck felt so weak and sore. One treatment involved me lying on my side to make sure my crushed lung was fully inflated. This was a worthy and sensible idea, except for the fact that when I lay on my side, the large draining tube inserted into my lung crunched on the broken bones. I made up my mind to jump out the window rather than endure this again. I begged the physio to stop. Ted, Helen and my brother Marcus appealed on my behalf, but their pleas were to no avail: I had to have the treatment.

Throughout the twenty-minute treatment I screamed and sobbed in agony as the machine did its thing with me. The family comforted me, making desperate promises of future pleasures to distract me. When at last I was released from the torture I realised Helen was crying and Ted and Marcus were drenched in perspiration. The next day I once again explained to the physio that I could not endure another treatment on my side. Her reply almost knocked me out of bed. 'Walk around instead, that's okay. Anyway, I've never seen anyone with as many rib breaks as you've got'.

I had a task. Here was something I *could* do! I was determined to walk! My children would accompany me: Helen would hold the pole with the drip, Ann the catheter bag, Ken would support me and last, but not least, Rob, like a bridesmaid, would hold the hem of my dressing-gown to stop me tripping over it. What a strange procession we must have made as I hobbled around the corridors with my retinue.

Around this time the registrar decided I needed tests to determine what was wrong with my eyes. Only partly clothed in an open hospital gown, with my right arm strapped up to my neck, my bottle of blood, my bottle of wee, the morphine drip and my eye-patch, I was wheeled past 50 waiting outpatients to wait my turn. Fascinated children peered up at me, asking, 'What's wrong with you?'

What could I say? Tears flooded my face from pain, fear and shame at being semi-naked in a public place. Miraculously, one of the mothers from my school was working at the desk. She found a blanket to cover my nakedness and moved my wheelchair into a side corridor for the long wait. The final straw came when the two students who eventually did the test spent all their time arguing if it was my left or right eye they were examining. This difficult question that could be answered if they had only stood beside me in the direction I was facing!

I also needed a brain scan. I was so terrified after so many tests that I pleaded with Ted to accompany me down to the x-ray department. I felt excruciatingly guilty about keeping him from work, yet I knew I just had to have him there. Just to move onto the x-ray table required extra pain-killing injections. I was put flat on the metal table in a brusque manner, every bone in my back shrieking in agony. My paralysed right arm had to be strapped to my body and in the haste of the whole process the broken bones in my clavicle were disconnected.

Having my head inserted into the narrow aperture for the scanning process made my brain go ballistic; I couldn't believe the fear and panic it caused. At the time it did not occur to me that the fear was due to the claustrophobia I now know I suffer. My brain must have registered being crushed in the car for 40 minutes while the Jaws of Life cut the metal around me. I was told not to worry because I had contact at all times with the technicians via a microphone. I endeavoured to remain still as directed over the microphone. I could see them chatting in the booth behind the glass walls. But it all got too much for me: I sobbed, screamed and pleaded into the microphone for someone to unstrap my shattered arm.

When I was eventually pulled out of the machine, exhausted, limp and almost unconscious, I asked why someone wouldn't help me. 'Oh, we turn off the microphone,' was the reply.

After two weeks of pain, noise, confusion and the bustle of the ward I felt certain I was about to go insane. I'd begged Ted constantly to try to get me transferred to another hospital where there was a single room, or to the empty single room next door. I had found out about this room when shuffling on a nurse's arm to the bathroom. I wanted that empty room more than anything I've ever wanted. I would stumble around the corridor and sit in the relative bliss of silence on seats near the lifts. I would hide in the tiny sitting-room and, when I was found, I would beg to sleep the night there on the floor. But this was all to no avail.

At last I realised that nobody would get me moved to the single room. Something snapped inside my head! No-one understood my predicament. Even Ted didn't realise I couldn't heal or improve in such a chaotic environment. I cracked. One day when I was in the bathroom I locked myself in and refused to come out until I could have the empty single room next door. Action! Ted was phoned and arrived very quickly.

As he put it, 'Even though in a damaged and desperate state, Chris produced the hat trick. Locking herself in the bathroom and refusing to leave till a solution was found led to the miraculous availability of a single room. Although it was vacated by a patient sent home for the weekend, once installed there was going to be a major altercation to get Chris out. Fortunately this was not needed.'

They say silence is golden. Never was silence more welcome.

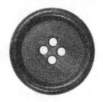

4.
In a room of my own

I want to be alone!

I learnt that the nursing staff had been reluctant to move me because I was so seriously ill and they didn't wish me to be isolated because they thought it would make me depressed. They thought the other patients would keep me company.

It took the family many trips to move all my flowers and cards from the ward. These things were concrete symbols of good wishes, they were also reminders of who I was.

Settled into my room of silence, I could start to mend.

The pain was still horrific three weeks after the accident. I had been able to get rid of the catheter, oxygen was only used some of the time, painkillers were still administered via my neck, and the physio visited regularly to put 'the pump' on my face to help keep my lungs inflated. In the morning a heroic effort was required to move my stiff body to the shower. To lift my back from the bed by using the knotted rope overhead took all my courage and strength. If someone had said, 'Your back has attached itself to the bed overnight,' I wouldn't have been surprised.

What an achievement it was when I could shower unaided. I would wobble my way to the bathroom and collapse in the shower cubicle. Sitting on the shower chair I would wrestle with pyjamas when it was time to remove them or put them on. The sensation of the warm water on my pain wracked body nearly pushed aside, for a fleeting second, the pain, terror, fear and bewilderment.

I could not lift my arms to put on my nightgown. Ann solved that problem with a pair of scissors. She split the necklines down to my waist and stitched on fastener ties of tape since my limbs would not obey and I couldn't work out how to do up buttons or how to put my legs in the leg holes. I would put on my clothes inside out. The nurses would have to redress me later, but still I tried.

I attempted to spend as much time as possible of each day propped up with pillows in a chair. It was drummed into me that movement was of the greatest importance to stop blood clots from forming and to hold the dreaded pneumonia at bay. Even when in bed I tried to keep my legs moving to supplement the regular injections to prevent clotting.

I had little appetite and no sense of smell or taste. When I chewed I would bite my lip or tongue, and the food would dribble out of my mouth, or I would choke and have to painfully cough. Numerous times the tray of food would be placed out of my reach. It would remain there unless a kindly hospital cleaner brought it nearer or put the straw in the box of Sustain so that I could have a drink. The kindness, empathy and sympathy of the cleaners were wonderful. I suppose no-one thought of feeding me and I couldn't think to ask for help even if I'd had the right words.

Ted was becoming increasingly worried about how little I ate, and one day he brought in an egg from home and used the microwave in the nurses' room to cook it. He didn't know how to cook using this method and he cooked the egg for eight minutes then fed it to me. They say love is blind, perhaps it's tasteless too, because I managed (just) to get it down to please him.

I felt such a nuisance to the nurses, who always seemed so hassled. I vividly remember one night being too ashamed or afraid to ring the bell to ask for a bedpan. With enormous pain I managed to pull off my bed-socks, thinking to use them for mopping up operations, only to realise that I didn't know what I'd do with the wet socks.

Days dragged on. Pain, clumsiness, bewilderment and difficulties dominated from the moment the bars around my bed were let down. I had to grit my teeth to pull on the knotted rope to get up to the sitting position, then I'd slowly shuffle to sit in a chair to have the pump and wait for Ted, as he popped in for a few minutes each morning on his way to work. I worried that he was looking so worn out. He looked so busy and hassled I did not dare ask him to stay. Visits from friends were hard because I found it so difficult to understand what they were talking about or find something to say to them.

I'd shuffle round the corridors on my constitutional walk and collapse from exhaustion afterwards. I was bitterly disappointed that I did not appear to be making progress.

Ted would call in again on his way home. As the night closed in I tried to stay awake, to put off the agony of the stiffening up process caused by being in bed. My brother Marcus had brought in a small portable television. I would sit propped up on my pillows in the chair straining to see and hear (after my episode in the ward I was paranoid about disturbing anyone!). I could not understand what was going on, but somehow it was company.

I'd need assistance to get into bed, and then the side bars would be pulled up. At times the thought of 'What if there is a fire?' made me realise how feeble, dependent and out of control I was. Even with heavy painkillers every few hours I was wracked in pain. Horrific technicolour nightmares emerged out of my pain.

During my fifth week in hospital the remaining tubes in my neck were removed. One evening, a short time after the removal of the tubes and the sticking plaster that had held them in place, I tried to tidy my hair before Ted was due to arrive. I noticed in the mirror that the right side of my neck was black. I painfully rubbed the area to try to remove the mark and then I asked a nurse to try shifting it with some methylated spirits. I was convinced that it was sticky stuff left by all the equipment and tubes, but the stain would not shift. I had no words to ask what it was. I could only wonder in my head, since gestures and pointing appeared to be my major way of communicating. Weeks later I realised it had been a bruise caused by the seat belt of the car when I was trapped and choking.

There had been some progress: I was now off oxygen, the painkilling injections had been superseded by medication. This actually meant I was in a lot more pain, but it was explained that I might become dependent on the injections if I continued on them. I could hobble about the passageways even if I missed doorways and walked into the door-jambs or walls by mistake. My balance was terrible: it was as if the floor was a heaving ship in high seas, but I yearned to go home, both for my sake and my family's. I was convinced that if only I could get home I might feel better. I overheard doctors talking amongst themselves. They were saying that they would not release me till I was walking well.

So I entered a new phase where I tried to pretend I was better than I was. I did endless rounds of the corridors; it was like walking the decks when I was 12 and my family went to England by ship. Every day I asked the doctor 'When can I go home?', but this request only seemed to instigate a lecture about going on to another hospital, a rehabilitation hospital. I had no clue what that meant. The only people I knew who were rehabilitated were soldiers, and I wasn't one, so I figured the doctor must have been mixed up.

During this time I suffered from incredible, vivid, technicolour 'dreams' (months later I learnt that this was epilepsy). Reality and unreality were intertwined. I had never experienced anything like it, but I could not tell anyone about it because of my difficulty communicating. I also had the sneaking suspicion that I had gone mad, and I didn't want other people to know. They wouldn't let me go home if I was insane!

So I fumbled, shuffled and stumbled my way around the corridors, determination on two wobbly legs — I'd walk my way out of the place! Doctors would promise escape the following day, only to produce another excuse for why I could not possibly go home when that day arrived. But eventually, seven weeks after the accident, I was told I could go home. What excitement!

Ken came to take me home. He carefully packed all my things into bags and managed to elegantly balance the wheelchair with me in it, my case, bags of cards and arrangements of flowers on our trip down in the lift and out into the bright winter sunshine.

For a short time Ken left me in the wheelchair, belongings piled nearby, and went to get the car. I was alone, helpless. But I was alive, the air was sweet, everything sparkled and shone, the mountains were a hazy blue smudge on the horizon. Behind me were the high dark walls of the hospital, looking like the tall walls of a castle. I shivered at the thought of the horror and pain contained within. A woman waiting beside me lit up a cigarette and I nearly screamed at her, 'Put it out! What about your poor precious lungs? You'll end up in there and you won't like that.'

But I didn't. I turned away, thankful and astonished at being outside in the fresh crisp air.

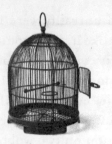

5.
Home among the gum trees

I've discovered that animals seem to understand.
I've discovered that sunshine on your back is fantastic.

Home. I'd never realised how much I loved our home perched among the gum trees on the top of a steep slope. The kids had the whole place sparkling and everywhere there were flowers from well-wishers. Daffodils from the bulbs I had planted two days before the accident swayed on their fragile stems in pots on the deck. How wonderful to be home. How incredible to leave home one day and not return for seven weeks.

Our black poodle, Steff, was beside himself with delight to see me. He bounded up to me and Ken had to grab him by the tail to stop him from knocking me over. Within a couple of minutes Steff seemed to sense and understand my pain. From then on he would follow me about calmly. If I sat down he would leap up beside me on my good left side. Most of the breaks to my ribs were on the right side, my clavicle was smashed and my right hand unworkable with fingers that could not move. I felt that my left side was better although my left hand was clenched into a ball and would not obey me and my left foot dragged when I walked. When I rested in bed Steff would lie on the floor beside me. For the next few months he hardly left my side.

I staggered around for an inspection. All the time a strange little cloud was following me about, inside and outside. It was good to be home but in some surreal, strange way it was, and was not familiar. I had escaped the labyrinth of hospital only to find home was yet another labyrinth.

My thoughtful family had constructed a slope of folded sleeping bags and pillows on my bed so that I could rest while being propped up. Oh, there's nowhere like your own bed, but it was frightening to be in so much pain.

I spent the day eagerly anticipating Ted's return from work that evening. At the dining-table that first evening home I looked around at members of my two-headed family with a measure of joy and pain. The girls cut up my food and I tried to feed myself with my fingers. I had trouble finding my mouth to poke in the food. I could taste nothing, I knocked over a glass of water, I spilt my food down my front, I choked and coughed. I couldn't follow or understand what they were talking about. Memories of happy meals, of my insistence on table manners swamped me. I stumbled off to bed. I felt stupid, wicked, guilty, clumsy and ugly.

And so me and my 'pain shadow' lived hand-in-hand. Everywhere I went it came also: in my back and ribs, clavicle and down my paralysed right arm. It was frightening pain. I couldn't sit up or move without being dumped by powerful waves of pain.

When I woke up in the mornings I was overwhelmed with panic as I tried to work out who I was, where I was, what was wrong with me and what day it was. It was like being lost in a labyrinth. This sense of bewilderment stayed with me all day until I gingerly crawled into bed at night, my senses dulled by painkillers and sleeping pills. The nights continued to be a time of terror, when I fought with the wild dragon of pain. Every three hours Ted would gently and carefully pull me upright using the sheepskin as a lifting band for spreading the pressure and to move me more evenly, so that I could take another painkiller.

Frequently my arm would go into spasm and I would scream until the pain slowly dissipated. My movements were very limited. Being carried caused unbearable pain. Getting into and out of bed was excruciating.

Early one morning I had a great deal of difficulty rousing Ted to pull me up so that I could take another painkiller. He moaned, 'I've just taken a sleeping pill to try to get some sleep'. That did it. I had spent so many agonised hours at night shaking with pain, hating to wake poor Ted to sit me up. There had to be another way. By swapping to the other side of the bed I discovered that I could force myself into a sitting position by pulling on the bottom sheet and pushing with my legs on the wall. What an achievement!

I spent my days wandering about the house, sitting and resting on a bed in the glassed-in room overlooking the valley. Ken cut back the tree-fern fronds so that I had a view of the bridge in the distance, the tree-covered slopes of Eltham, the artist's colony Montsalvat and the blue mountains beyond. This scene would vary according to the eye I was using.

In the hospital the doctors had explained that double vision was frequently the result of a head injury. Sometimes the eyes righted themselves, sometimes they could be operated on if they had stabilised. However, the doctors were fairly certain that in a few years' time, even with operations, I would only have a 'keyhole' of normal vision in the centre of my gaze, with double vision above and below. Without the patch, everyone had two heads, three or four eyes. There would be two spoons where there was only one. The doctors suggested I patch one eye to block out the second image, alternating right and left eye. Depending on which eye was patched the colours were different. The world tilted on different angles and at night the double moon seen through the glass ceiling, or double lights from street lights, would move and wander up and down through the landscape. Months later Ann made me a variety of eye patches to match my different clothes.

Ted's activities were heavily curtailed as he spent his evenings watching videos with me and reading to me. According to him, 'it was obvious that she didn't follow storylines but this at least kept her in contact with external stimulation and thoughts. Her melancholy was a consistent and extensive; something never seen before in such a positive person.'

Helen remembers some 'terrible fights as Mum was very, very angry at not being able to do things for herself, humiliated that her children and husband whom she believed she should look after, had to look after her. On a number of occasions I would find her sobbing and she would say she couldn't go on and that life in such pain was not worth living.'

Birds constantly visited the feeding tray out in the tree, and at times the bare limbs of the witch elm would be festooned with a dozen currawongs, all singing their mournful song. They moved on to make way for a family of four kookaburras, and later the amusing antics of two huge baby magpies and their parents. One certainly can't feel lonely with animals about. They gave me some comfort during the long dull days. I used to lie for hours staring at them, my mind blanked out by pain and drugs.

The kindness of my children was overwhelming. After Ted went to work in the morning Helen and Ann would do their individual tasks for me. It became apparent that the day would not seem so long if I could delay getting up for as long as possible. But with stiffness and pain, staying in bed was difficult. Helen would come downstairs to the bedroom, hop on to the bed and try to distract me with conversation. I was very puzzled that I could not follow or understand what she said and would make what I thought were appropriate noises. It was crazy — I could hear the words but not understand them. I could not remember a second later what she had said, or what topics she had been discussing.

Then Helen would help me to sit up and I would gingerly heave myself out of bed to totter to the shower. My head would spin, I would overbalance and slip, I would go to grab the soap and miss it, I would have the greatest difficulty remembering if my hair was wet because I had washed it or was about to wash it. Was this because of my terrible double vision? I found it strange that I had absolutely no concept of the time the shower had taken. Sometimes I felt as if I had been showering or dressing for a split second, other times as if I had been doing the same action for half a lifetime.

Ann, meanwhile, would have put out a tracksuit, socks and so forth in readiness for the marathon struggle of the day called getting dressed. Luckily Rob had a couple of track suits I could wear. I was like a child. I wore the clothes Ann put out. I never thought of asking the girls to buy me some track suits of my own. Perhaps we thought I'd be better in a week or so!

With my right arm paralysed and in a sling, even putting on my socks presented excruciating difficulties.

My left hand was not too nifty at doing up buttons so a tracksuit was better than shirt and jeans. It felt more normal to have the girls do up the zip of the tracksuit for me than do up my buttons.

And so I'd struggle on while the girls prepared breakfast. I ate to try to overcome the floaty, nauseous feeling, hoping that my lack of taste, smell and appetite didn't show. In those early days I started to realise that being a convincing actress was going to be of great importance in making those about me feel more comfortable.

I could not express the strange things happening to me and around me; all my energy and resources were taken up just trying to endure the pain and live, move and eat. This was a time just to exist, to try to get my poor ribs to heal. The head injuries and what they entailed would not be looked into for many weeks.

But I was so puzzled because I didn't know what 'sit' meant if someone said 'sit down' and I couldn't recognise a glass or a brush unless I saw the object in a certain position. It was weird. At the time no-one explained to me that my confusion was caused by my head injury. The damage my brain had suffered meant that my short-term memory had gone, so I couldn't remember something told to me five seconds earlier. My long-term memory was mostly intact, which explained why I remembered my family and parts of my home. However, I'd forgotten where light switches were, and couldn't remember where the tap was in the garden. Because we'd altered the layout of the kitchen ten years previously I looked for drawers, articles and cupboards where they had been over a decade ago.

Later I obtained a publication put out by Headway Victoria, which explained the results of a bad bang on the head. To learn that difficulty with motor ability and control, balance and coordination, and lack of sensations like touch, pain, temperature, taste and smell, and sensitive hearing are all legitimate problems after head injury was a tremendous relief. If only I had been given this information in hospital, I would not have felt so confused and worried that I had gone mad, or that if only I tried harder I would be able to see or understand or walk or talk properly. I didn't tell anyone how I felt because my short-term memory loss meant that I didn't remember! I was also loath to complain about what I considered 'small' things.

Lack of depth perception caused many problems when I moved about. Our home has three levels with the bedroom on the lowest level. I knew that the ground was at the end of my legs, but when it came to the act of placing my foot on the ground, it seemed to be miles away. These visual and spatial problems made it difficult going downstairs, for example. While I felt a little foolish, holding on to an old broomstick helped me whenever I had to go downstairs.

I found out that a head injury can also result in an inability to accurately interpret visual information. So while I knew the word hairbrush, and I could open the bathroom drawer to find it, I could not recognise it when it was there in front of me. I also had great difficulty reading facial expressions, which compounded my feelings of isolation and guilt.

I learnt I was not being unreasonable or crazy in the hospital when I found the noise driving me nuts. With hindsight the scan that showed the fracture to my skull and the double vision should have made it obvious that I needed peace and quiet in order to mend. If I had been sent to a ward for head injuries, perhaps my recovery and rehabilitation would have been different. But we were not to know the extent of my injuries at the time.

I also discovered from the Headway Kit that perceptions can frequently mislead a head-injured person and thus they may respond inappropriately. One-sided neglect of my brain explained why I left part of my dinner on the left side of the plate — I didn't know it was there! Months later at rehab, I was taught to move my head to scan my plate or the passageway I was walking down. This prevented more bumps and bruises.

At various times of the day I would hold court amid my bower of flowers in the glassed-in room overlooking the valley. Ann would be busy brewing endless cups of coffee and putting out new cups. My visitors would chat among themselves. I felt strange and detached, as if I was there but not there. I had to act out my part as I could not follow or understand the conversations, so I switched on a sort of automatic pilot. People were so kind — visiting, bringing flowers, food and friendly words — but inside me festered a secret sore. I must be a bad and horrid person because I felt so cold and numb, and not nearly grateful or thankful enough for the kindness heaped on me. I felt so helpless, so alone, so strange.

It was not until four years later when I saw an advertised lecture about shell-shock that I came to understand about post-traumatic stress disorder. I attended the lecture and learnt that symptoms of this disorder include feeling numb and dazed. You feel depersonalised, as if your brain is outside your body, and time seems unreal. You don't know who you are and experience despair, hopelessness, denial and guilt.

My body felt as if it was shaking inside. I had difficulty concentrating. My short-term memory was terrible. I felt no-one knew or understood how I felt. I was snappy and aggressive. Little things blew out of all proportion. Day and night, dreams constantly returned me to the horrific scene. I became emotionally numb and tried to avoid thoughts, feelings and activities. I no longer took pleasure in things that previously had caused me pleasure. I felt totally cut off from everyone, and didn't see a future worth having. Frequently a noise or movement would startle me so badly that I'd shake with fright, and my heart would palpitate. Later I'd feel totally dumb because of my overreaction.

If only someone had talked to me about post-traumatic stress disorder, and helped me to understand and express what I was experiencing! If it had been explained that such feelings of disorientation and frustration were normal for someone who has been involved in an accident, I might not have experienced so much guilt and stress. Information, psychological support, crisis intervention, and emotional first-aid were needed to assist me to address my depression, social agoraphobia, chronic pain and panic, not to mention being house-bound and experiencing marital disharmony and difficulties with employment. It has been suggested that 50 per cent of those who suffer post-traumatic stress remain chronic sufferers after ten years.

Things were hard on the people around me, too. As Helen puts it:

> 'In the early weeks when she came home from hospital Mum was extremely irrational, frustrated and downright nasty. She annoyed us all as she repeated herself, was over-anxious about our safety and generally found it impossible to relax. Mum was not like this before her accident and while I can try to rationalise the problems she has to cope with, her behaviour caused friction. At times Mum dwelt upon the man who hit her car. She became upset and often mentioned the man who changed her life. When she was extremely distressed I could find little to comfort her as I found it hard to cope myself. I mourned for the woman my mother was, but I'm determined to help her make the best of what she was left with.'

In retrospect I can't fathom why I did not ask my doctor about these things. I can only suppose I couldn't reason sufficiently to put the symptoms all together and realise there was something really wrong. Perhaps it was because in my mind they all added up to one fact: I had gone mad! In isolation, the difficulties seemed like small things, and I hated to whinge. Hope springs eternal, and one always thinks, 'Tomorrow will be different, I won't forget or break things or be dumb. I'll try harder and beat it.'

As dusk approached each evening I would feel fear and terror start to bubble up uncontrollably. The night that meant fear of pain would come again. The minutes would creep by so slowly. I would hear the clatter of the children preparing dinner and silently weep. On a tape I recorded:

> *'I feel so frustrated I could go screaming mad. There have been so many weeks of pain, confusion and dependence. At times I think it would have been simpler on my family (and me) if I'd died, if the blackness had swallowed me and they could be rebuilding and getting on with their lives. At other times I'm just so thankful to have been miraculously spared.*
>
> *Everyone says how well I'm doing, which means that they don't even have a glimpse of the agony, indignity and horror. How can life ever be sweet again? Did I ever value each second, each blade of grass? Where has my enormous store of hope and joie de vivre gone? Life seems so bleak. Will I never have that glorious bubbly feeling that life's wonderful again? That man has destroyed more than my body, he has twisted and crushed my spirit, like my twisted and crushed car. I have lost me.'*

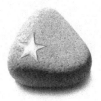

6.
Spitting chips!

In the wee small hours does Mr X ever think of the woman he hit?
Does he resolve 'I must take more care.'
Or has the whole episode passed from his mind?

My unknown hero's hand, voice, dragging and rescuing me
From the beckoning black void of Death.
And I've never even seen his face.

After I had been home a few weeks, the man who had helped me when I was trapped in the car rang to inquire how I was getting on. He had rung Ted while I was in hospital to check on my progress. Peter had been driving in the other direction. He saw the accident and stopped immediately to see what he could do. He noticed that I was having trouble breathing so he smashed the passenger window and managed to get the seat belt from around my neck where it was choking me. (This explained the terrible black bruising on my neck.) He asked passers-by to ring the police and ambulance. This quick-thinking and practical man then stayed with me for the 40 minutes it took to cut me free of the wreckage. How fortunate he was passing by at that moment!

A thought constantly nagged in my mind when I was convalescing: an overwhelming desire to meet my hero, the man behind the voice in the echo in my mind, 'You've been clipped, you'll be okay'. I had to meet him.

And so it was that one of my early trips in a car was to visit this kind man. Peter lived only a few kilometres from the accident site. He was a resourceful and practical person, and endeavoured to shrug off his stopping to help me as nothing. Ted and I were acutely aware that but for Peter I might not be here, or I might be in a nursing home. Just knowing what Peter had done for me seemed very important. I must confess that I was a tiny bit disappointed that seeing him brought back no memory of the time he'd stayed with me, although perhaps deep in my subconscious there was something about his voice I found very calming.

It was only after quite some time had passed and we had met on several occasions that Peter came to tell me how the whole incident had affected him. Apparently after assisting me he went home and had a stiff whisky and said to his wife that he didn't think I would make it.

Why didn't the man who had hit me ring to find out if I was dead or alive? I overheard Ted telling someone on the phone that the police had told him that man had driven across the road to get a quote to have his car fixed. (Later the police prosecutor noted that the smash repairer's records supported this.) I would lie in bed in the small hours crying silently in pain, cursing the man who had so carelessly ruined my life. I would fantasise about arriving at his house and pouring red nail polish, a symbol of my blood, down the windscreen of his precious car. How dare he go about as if nothing had happened when he was personally responsible for injuring and crushing another human being?

My bitterness grew, fuelled by people asking, 'What happened to the man who hit you?' Of course the answer was: nothing. He eats and sleeps, and life goes on as usual for him. 'I'll show him,' I thought. It was then that the idea to record my experiences surfaced. Rather than daydream about catching a taxi to his house to disfigure his car, I would record my experiences in a book to let him know what he had done.

A cake of 'Paris' soap finally led me to realise I couldn't let him destroy my life. One day, a year after the accident, as I was using Ted's birthday gift of Paris soap, I told myself how lucky I was that I could have this occasional luxury. It was then I realised that hating 'Mr.X' was a luxury I could no longer afford if I was going to conserve my strength to get better. The bad, black days filled with hate were gradually, oh so gradually, overtaken by days when I didn't curse him. After a couple of years things had changed so dramatically that I got to the stage of actually worrying about him being forced go to jail, until a friend pointed out how unlikely this was. These days a week can pass without me thinking or saying his name.

When I was on my feet a little more Helen, Ann, Ken and Rob cooked a special Sunday lunch and Mum, Dad and my brother Marcus came to meet Peter, his wife Gaye and their two gorgeous kids. At the time I must have still been pretty wonky, but I can remember a warm glow that was not just from the roaring fire in the fireplace.

If I had hand-picked a hero I could not have done better. As well as being practical in helping me at the accident Peter was the best witness. In a calm unruffled way he was able to tell the police exactly what had happened. Peter helped to banish the grey clouds of anger and gloom. He was my symbol of good overcoming bad.

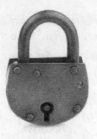

7.
Stuck in a glass box

I feel like an alien.
I have to drum up enthusiasm to open cards, read letters, express appreciation.
Am I still a member of the human race?

Life went on. The days and weeks passed slowly, so slowly. I could just hold a pen to sign the thank you letters the kids prepared. I could also shuffle up our drive as far as our mail box, a very adventurous thing to do. I would try to help the kids by unpacking the top of the dishwasher on to the bench; I couldn't put the knives and forks in the drawer because I would forget which section they belonged to. I would wander from the sitting room to the glassed in room, and I would lie on the bed and say 'Arrrr' — proof that I was alive and I could do something even if it was only making a noise.

Without a sense of taste or smell I didn't enjoy eating although every hour or so the kids would bring me a cut orange to eat. They had read in Tony Moore's book *Cry of the Damaged Man* how he had a craving for oranges after he had a horrific car accident. If he ate oranges, maybe I would like them too! I could not see properly or concentrate enough to read. My ears couldn't stand noise of a talking book or music. I think my first stirring of a wisp of happiness was warmth: the feeling of holding warm coffee in a fine, old cup in my hand; rays of sunshine on my back; the warmth of the love and care of my family.

Kind folk continued to faithfully visit, bringing good cheer, flowers and food. I was still numb inside. I'd say 'It's fantastic!' 'Marvellous!' 'How interesting!' 'Look forward to it!' 'Fascinating!' 'Wow!' But the words didn't mean a thing. It was as if I was locked in an invisible glass box, totally isolated from the rest of the world. The door-bell continued to ring at dusk for months as florists delivered bouquets from friends and families of girls I had taught up to a decade before. People were so kind.

I was fortunate to have a wonderful GP and physio. They visited me regularly at home for the first few weeks. When I was able to travel the family would take me to appointments and months later, I would go by taxi. Hugh, my GP, strengthened both my body and my spirit. Hugh first came to see me one sunny afternoon when I had been home a week. He spoke of car-racing, his passion. He said 'It is up to you whether you recapture your life, whether you're out of the race of life or not. The choice is yours, whether you allow this to ruin your life or whether you fight, struggle and work to get back in the car and get back in the race.' He spoke with admiration of racing drivers who'd had their bodies but not their spirits smashed.

Hugh arranged for me to have physiotherapy regularly and Philip, my physio, would visit, sometimes as late as 11pm, to help me get my paralysed right arm moving. He explained to Ted how I needed a pulley with a sling attached for my right arm. I could then place my wrist in it and pull on the pulley with my left hand, thus lifting the immobile arm. Ever resourceful, Ted fitted up a pulley arrangement from a beam in our bedroom so that I could exercise my motionless arm several times a day.

I did no housework, shopping or cooking. I could not read or follow the correct line on a page, or the plot in a book or newspaper. I could not thread a needle or find the holes to do tapestry, which I used to enjoy so much. I could not see to hold a brush to paint and watercolour painting had been a joy to me. I could not go for walks because of my lack of balance and poor depth perception. I could not tell where the ground was and my feet looked like they were ten feet away. It was weird not knowing where my feet or my mouth were. I had the attention span of a gnat. I did not know what day it was and even when I was told, I'd forget a second later.

Ted, the kids and Mum and Dad tried to think up ways to help me overcome my disabilities. They wrote lists for me: 'Today is Monday. At 11am there is a doctor's appointment, you will need to be ready at 10.30am.'

For many weeks Helen and Ann mothered me, putting out clothes and helping me dress. After some time I tried to organise myself. They would help by making lists so that I would remember to do things that I used to do automatically: get up, shower, put on socks, undies, check that my clothes were not inside out, start buttoning my shirt from the bottom button and move up the shirt, eat breakfast, take my pills, go and lie in the glass room. Eat lunch at 12.30, and so on.

I had panic attacks when the phone rang, so they wrote in clear letters on a piece of paper: Pick up the phone, say 'Hello, this is Christine, Who's calling please?' If I needed to ring someone I wrote down the points of the conversation on paper and read out the questions and answers. If I didn't do this I would totally forget why I had contacted the person.

I think one of the biggest disappointments was that I simply couldn't tolerate music, something I had always had a passion for. Nor could I listen to the radio or television because they really hurt my ears. I could not work in the garden because of my lack of coordination and balance, and I could not understand the conversations of my family or friends. With no sense of taste or smell I couldn't even drown my sorrows with food or drink.

For months I cried daily. I wanted to die, to escape from this me that wasn't me. For over a year I couldn't do something as simple as ask for bread in a shop without crying. I wept with despair, frustration, pain, disappointment, jealousy and desire to be normal. I cried because no-one seemed to understand what life was like for me. I was fortunate I didn't get 'face rot' from having a wet face much of the time! Tears were never far from the surface. I cried not at the drop of a hat, but unexpectedly, in the middle of conversations with family, friends and strangers. It was embarrassing and perplexing.

I was so fortunate to have the kids and Ted. Helen had very early on realised that I would have to depend on them for everything.

> 'As a family it became obvious that Mum's quality of life relied upon us working as a unit and thus each of us did our utmost to support her. I have high respect for my siblings due to the many sacrifices they made, especially my two brothers who were such assistance to Mum typing on the computer; Ken for being a tireless chauffeur and Rob for the encouragement he so obviously gave her. Ann looked after Mum and ran the household for six months and did not seek employment.'

Ken also realised that things had to be changed to accommodate my needs.

> 'Being strong-willed, Mum was constantly attempting things that were clearly beyond her ability. Often we would find her in the garden or laundry weeping with pain and frustration after trying to prune the roses or hang up washing. Our supervisory role was now greatly increased to prevent her combination of physical injury and impaired judgment damaging her further, and someone had to keep a constant eye on her.

> For at least four months after coming home from hospital she took the almost total attention of my father and two sisters in feeding, bathing and comforting. An image of her doing arm-strengthening exercises, hysterical and screaming from pain, will always be in my mind. She would lie in a bed in the glass living-room and weep with pain and frustration and almost from shame — being unable to walk properly or even sit showed a weakness

she would never allow. This strength of character is what has driven her recovery, though this same stubbornness has also caused her mental suffering.'

Several months passed after the accident, before acceptance really hit me. It was a Saturday night. The family all sat in front of a warm, crackly fire to watch a good video. I supported myself with painkillers, a hot-water bottle and pillows, and managed to escape for a brief time and forget that I was now different. Then the video ended and realisation hit me, as if for the first time: 'I am a damaged person, life is not the same'. This realisation opened up another thought: 'I must try to recapture life, I must get back into the world and amongst people'.

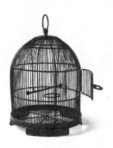

8.
Out of my glass box and into the world

*My hands trip, my feet trip, my thoughts trip, my tongue trips, my brain trips.
I trip therefore I am.*

One Saturday morning I asked Ted to take me to a large shopping complex not far from home. I wanted to be out amongst people again. I quaked and shook, and, feeling like St George off to do battle with the dragon, I carefully walked along the walls of the shops.

I had been locked away from the world for so long it felt amazing to be out and about again, to see so many people and so many children. After some time I noticed a little girl looking at me. 'Now are you from school? Do I know you? Have I taught you?' I asked myself. I smiled at her and she smiled back. It seemed strange and weird — all the children I passed smiled at me, some even craning their necks as they passed. It wasn't until we passed a mirror that I realised that with my eye patch they must have thought I was a lady pirate!

This brief glimpse of the world made me desperate to see my students at school again. How I missed school and the students.

I had to work out when to go and when to get ready — an almost insurmountable task just to organise a visit — my third trip out of home. The morning of the visit arrived. I was sitting up in bed howling with pain when the phone on the other side of the bed started to ring. I couldn't lean across to pick up the receiver and I was in too much pain to heave myself out of bed to shuffle round to the other side to answer it, so I had no option but to let it ring out.

The dressing and getting ready accomplished, Ken helped me as I gingerly and painfully got into the car. We got to school to find it deserted. Not a pupil or teacher in sight! That unanswered phone call had been from school to say that everyone would be away for the day on an excursion. Later that week we did a repeat of the trip and I did manage to catch up with 'my' kids, a wonderful but painful experience, as they all hugged me.

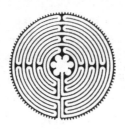

9.

Rehab: Trapped in a different labyrinth

And we all thought 'It couldn't happen to me'.
At the Rehabilitation Hospital we all walk funny,
We all talk funny, we all think funny.
But it's not funny!

Small Talk
A bit like a bunch of brides discussing their big day.
But instead of attendants we discussed witnesses,
Instead of clothes the pain,
Instead of the groom, the other party.

Why?
I am innocent
I am innocent
I am innocent
What did I do?

Three months after the accident my GP, Hugh, decided it was time that I went to see a neurologist. Ken and Ann drove me into the city which seemed an amazing surreal world, familiar yet unfamiliar. Ann walked with me from the car to the building. I fumbled all the way, shaking, afraid, feeling so weird, floaty and different. Was this the same city I had once felt so at home in? I felt an outsider, an interloper in this new world.

The neurologist said I should be assessed for the extent of my head injuries. I was referred to a psychologist at a well-known rehabilitation hospital. On my first visit I completed the tests in a total daze. I cannot express my horror and amazement when I could not compute simple sums, the sort I had spent hours every week doing with my students. I was given other tests similar to the ones I used to give at school, but I couldn't concentrate long enough to even finish the exercises. I could only just cope with being alive, and that was all. Moving and concentrating for short bursts for the intensive testing was very difficult. A week or so earlier it would have been totally impossible.

I then began three half-days of rehabilitation a week with occupational therapy, speech therapy, a visit to the psychologist and group balance classes. The program seemed like a sensible way to tackle my problems. I could sleep each afternoon as I was still experiencing extreme exhaustion. On the other two days when I was not at the hospital, I visited the physio. These visits required a car journey of 20 minutes each way, either with one of the kids driving me or a taxi ride, a wait, and treatment that was frequently painful. Many times I would sob all the way home in the taxi. What a schedule to stick to! I was exhausted from all the terrifying taxi travel, bewildered from trying to find my way about, and worn out from all the never-ending pain.

I still had no concept of time, and would be full of unreasonable panic, expecting to be late for the appointment. So I would start getting ready at 9am for the noon arrival of the taxi to take me to the rehabilitation hospital. Ann would help to organise my clothes in the morning, but being alone in the house when the family went off for the day, I had to muddle through myself. I would eat lunch at 10am and be ready for the taxi, then I would worry why it was late, stumbling about the house in fear. I would be exhausted when it finally arrived on time. To actually sit in a car required a superhuman effort because I was sure that I would be in another accident. By the time we arrived at the hospital I would be shaking so much it was hard to walk in the front door.

The moment I stepped into the corridor of the hospital it was as though the filters on my eyes fell off, revealing reality. At home I could stumble, couldn't say what I wanted, repeat myself and it was just me being a bit strange. But put me in the midst of other head-damaged people and the reason I was the way I was became apparent. Perhaps we have a little antennae inside our heads that pick up the vibe so that we can recognise people who are like us.

There was the handsome young lawyer who wanted to hear from the hoons who'd come over the hill on the wrong side of the road and smashed into his vehicle; the young chap with little face or voice left who would weep, wanting to hear from the person who had done this to him; the woman who'd run off the road and into a tree, killing her husband, and somehow seemed lucky to have kangaroos to blame!

In the smoke-filled tea-room at the hospital I was interested to hear my query 'Who did this to me?' echoed by so many other people. We must have some innate desire to have justice done and for the people who cause pain to others to say they're sorry.

Many of my fellow patients were so innocent they made me cry, their stories so ghastly it was like suddenly finding myself in the middle of a horror movie. To think I had spent my life blissfully unaware that this nightmare world, this labyrinth that existed yet was hidden away from the 'normal' world.

Snatches of conversation would penetrate my thoughts while I was sitting in the tea-room: 'I got squashed in my car', 'They went through a red light', 'Kangaroos on the road', 'A stolen car chased by police', 'On the wrong side of the road', 'I've been here seven months', 'It happened a year ago', 'Gee I'm working to talk good!'. My heart bled for all of them. I was appalled at what innocent people in our society have to endure.

Perhaps the cruellest part of rehab for me was picking up my fellow patients feelings of fear, pain and hopelessness. Somehow, being aware of the suffering of others so similar to my own, to hear of their obviously unattainable hopes and dreams, made me wonder if I was as unrealistic as them. I shuddered at the thought.

There was also opportunity to observe other patients during group activities and I travelled home in the taxi run with the same people each session. I was at the end of the hour-long drop-off journey. One of my fellow travellers had been coming to rehab for five years, which amazed me. I naïvely thought that everyone would be better in that time. He'd had his accident on his motorbike. I was even more amazed when, one day on our trip home, he said, 'Good day for a ride. The sun's coming out, there's a bit of wind, freedom. Shame my artificial hip stops me riding.'

The entire rehab experience was so utterly new to me; I had absolutely nothing in my personal experience to relate it to. I felt just like Alice in Wonderland. Did Lewis Carroll write his book as an analogy of what it is like to have head injuries? The similarities are too close for comfort! Alice fell down a rabbit hole. She passed many curious things on the way down but was unable to stop to look, or understand what was happening. Alice's fall was down a tunnel towards darkness. There was light at the end of my tunnel. Like Alice I was shut up inside myself, like a folding telescope, in terrifying agony. Thoughts like 'Who am I?' formed in my mind. Like Alice said when she met the caterpillar, 'I'm afraid I can't explain myself, because I'm not myself'. This swearing, unhelpful, pain-racked person who could not see, walk or talk properly, this bumbling idiot child who had to be looked after by her children was not me. I felt wicked. I felt nobody understood.

Rehab had its good and bad points. It was very comforting when the doctor showed me the scans of my brain and pointed out where fluid had drained through the crack in my skull. Seeing 'proof' was so important. Two people from rehab were particularly helpful — the speech therapist (I saw her twice, she was kind and empathetic) and appeared to understand my condition, and Fran, who helped me return to work, showed great empathy and understanding.

I learnt to scan by turning my head from side to side — thus seeing the whole rather than just part of the opening — before going through doorways, or going down passages, which helped reduce bruising. Rehab gave me a reason to get out of the house and it gave me hope that the experts would fix me. But I found the judgmental approach of all the tests most upsetting. In the past I'd always succeeded in any test I'd attempted so I was acutely aware of all my inability. I could not understand the purpose of much that happened to me in rehab. Perhaps the experts tried to explain but I couldn't comprehend. I suspect pictures or diagrams would have made more sense to me than words.

It was at rehab I realised you cannot learn from someone who does not appear to like or value you. Some judgments made by the physios were incorrect and presumptuous. For example, when I inquired about whether a walking stick might help me, I was told that I was too young to have a stick, and anyway, I would get dependent on it and not want to give it up. I believed the experts and fumbled on as directed. However, after I left rehab I found that using a broomstick at home and later a walking stick helped me balance and to judge distance going down stairs. A stick gave me confidence when walking so I had less falls and people didn't perceive me as a drunk. A stick became a vital tool that helped me cope. I am cross that so much of my rehab involved being taught to walk along the street touching fences or shop windows instead of using a stick!

One day at rehab I actually ganged up with some bikies against the physio. My mates and I were doing some exercises around a tree trunk. The young physio appeared to have no idea how silly, futile and difficult the task was for us. If only he had explained what we were doing and why we were doing it! I'd never defied authority in my life but his 'them' and 'us' mentality made me rebel. We made fun of him and were quite bad-mannered. Afterwards although I felt shocked at myself because I'd behaved badly and disobeyed someone for the first time in my life, I found I really didn't care.

I'd also be overcome by the plight of my fellow patients at unexpected times. Once when I was sitting in occupational therapy an eighteen-year-old man was wheeled in. We waited together in silence. I said hello and asked him how he was. His answer and the poignancy of the moment shattered me, 'Me smell, me taste, me talk, me thoughts — no good. Me mate, he was on his L's, he was doing wheelies.' And then he was wheeled away. Several months later I found myself once again waiting with this young guy. He was out of his wheelchair and I commented about how good it was that his legs were better. 'Oh, it wasn't me legs,' was his reply, 'It was me head. I'd forgotten how to walk.'

Balance classes were traumatic. Imagine six damaged human beings swaying, faltering and falling, trying to catch a ball. One day the old man I was throwing the ball to teetered and nearly fell. The young man in the corner kept eagerly saying to the physio 'See me catch, Coach, I'm doing good, Coach!' The scarred woman in her twenties sat rocking, it was a bad day for her, and she kept saying, 'I don't want to be here, I want to go home'. The same thought sat behind the tears in my eyes as I looked at them. We all had the 'branding mark': three small puncture scars on our necks from tubes inserted when we were in intensive care. If a Martian were to come into the room it might seem that our brains and our balance had been sucked out by some cruel Dracula.

I worked with greater determination on my balance exercises when I was at home. In the sunshine and with the dog for company I spent hours wobbling my way along the paving cracks in the drive. This was my individual program: I felt some ownership in it, and I wanted to prove something by doing it. This contrasted sharply with trying to fit into a balance group session at the hospital.

In retrospect I know I needed lots of explanations and reasons for doing things in rehab. Most of the time I was paralysed with pain and longing for life as it had been, all the while being distracted by the amazing mental 'trips', the crazy happenings that were wilder than Alice's world. When I told the rehab experts about it they did not appear to understand. I was very disappointed when my mental strangeness was not explained. Later I was to discover it was epilepsy. At the time I just felt even more crazy and troublesome.

Looking back, many things could have assisted me at this stage of recovery. I desperately needed to talk to someone to help me cope with the loathing and hatred I felt towards the man who had done this to me. I needed help to deal with the changes in my life, to understand what my husband and family were thinking. I needed to be asked 'What do you want? What would be most helpful to you?' instead of doing tests, being judged, and told what I needed. Having a say would have empowered me.

I badly needed a sufferer's manual to help me make sense of the situation, to realise that what I was going through was normal. I needed encouragement rather than the implied criticism I felt from many of the rehab team. Deep down I knew I had a long way to go, so an explanation on why progress would be slow would have been beneficial. I was told that most of my recovery would occur during the first six months, then, there would be slow recovery until two years after the accident. That would be it.

My GP, Hugh, said he believed I would continue to improve for five years. As it turned out, I feel I made the most helpful progress in recapturing my life in the fifth year. I can remember my panic and consternation as the six-month, then two-year time barriers passed. The despair I felt, that I would be like this for the rest of my life!

I needed help to deal with the loss and grief. I'd lost myself, my ability to be the mother and wife I had been. I'd lost my career, my freedom and my ability to drive. Even shopping for the family's food was an almost impossible task. I needed to have post-traumatic stress and head injury explained to me, *so that I could understand*. I did not want to be told I was lucky I wasn't more badly hurt or dead!

I didn't want to forget. I needed to try to make sense of this crazy world, to remember and mourn.

I needed desperately to hear from another Alice who had been down the rabbit hole and survived. I wanted to be told that it was OK to feel frightened and confused. Someone who has sat at the top of the rabbit hole and had a picnic, even if they've peered down, taken photos and studied it, is not as helpful as someone who has fallen down that long, scary hole.

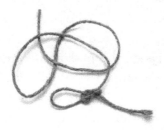

10.
The more you do the more you see your problems

'Chris, I've told you time and time again not to put gin on your cereal in the morning!'
I've never touched a drop yet I'm 'drunk' all the time!

I've discovered that slower can be faster.
I've discovered that frustration can take all my life energy.
I've discovered that keeping a diary can let you see progress.

It was now four months since the accident. I struggled and pushed myself to get better. I was absolutely determined to return to school for fourth term. But I was so slow and dim, whereas the 'old' me had been on the ball and done everything at whirlwind pace. In spite of wearing tracks on the drive doing my balance exercises, and wearing out the carpet on the stairs practising stepping up with one foot, across with the other foot then down with the other foot, my progress seemed almost non-existent.

I tried to teach myself the concept of time: everything I did, I timed. I'd guess how long it would take to do something or walk somewhere then I'd time myself. This was quite difficult because of my problem with numbers — I had lost my one-to-one correspondence. I found an analogue clock much more useful in trying to gauge the passing of time because I had the face of the clock to show me how much time had passed. I wrote down everything I did, and how long it took me, so I didn't forget. This helped me plan a little more efficiently. No longer was I ready at 9am for a 1pm appointment, instead I'd be ready at 10.30am! I changed from being an invalid who did nothing all day as I gradually started to do things again. It was then that the breadth and depth of my difficulties became apparent.

I tried to help the family by packing and unpacking the top section of the dishwasher on to the bench. I had a smashing time! With the eye-patch on I would ignore my left side and send things flying so they smashed or smashed into other things for double smashings. Without the eye-patch I would put things on the wrong image of the bench (in the air), again with smashing results. Each week there would be a pile of broken bowls, plates, glasses and vases by the rubbish bin.

My eyes were driving me crazy. I was afraid to constantly cover only one eye, because I was told this would lead to more long-term balance and vision problems. Clutching at straws, I tried patching alternate eyes on alternate days. This meant I'd have days when I couldn't walk straight. It was eerie seeing different colours with each eye, and if I coughed or sneezed in the dark I'd see flashing lights where none existed. Watching television without the patch meant double images: one set on an angle overlapping the other, and once again, the colours differed depending on the eye. If I looked at a page of a book with one eye it was green, with the other, cream — which was the real colour? I became fixated on the fact that I didn't know what the real colour was. I felt frustrated and frightened because I didn't know what was 'true' any more.

My eyes had been assessed after the accident in the hospital and later during a visit to the neurologist. Eventually I was referred to an eye surgeon. It was the moment I'd been waiting for. I'd been patient; I'd waited months for my eyes to settle down, *now* I could get them fixed. The surgeon took one look my pirate patch and said 'get that patch off and leave it off. Your eyes can't work together if you have a patch. Your eyes have to stop changing.' I stuffed my patch in my pocket and fumbled for the door. Thus started two nightmare months where I went patchless. Down the stairs, falter, fall, double moving images everywhere. I was shattered. I had to try to survive in this hideous, tilting, moving world, and I had been told in rehab not to use a stick.

Unexpectedly and amazingly, my sense of smell returned. I began to depend on touch for my sense of reality. Even the soles of my feet started to send me messages. I began to feel things with my hands — groping things I passed, embarrassingly, even people. My foot felt or tapped to feel where there were gutters or steps, and I limped as I still couldn't control my left side properly. I walked with my legs far apart, as if I'd just spent a day on a horse. A physio explained that I was doing this automatically to try to get more balance. I felt clumsy, ungainly, ugly and slow. I also experienced sensations of floating. It was all very weird.

Daily the phone calls would come from Mum and Dad. Dad was a great reader and had a deep interest in 'the head' (he'd been a pioneer in the hearing-aid field). He would have numerous suggestions: 'Chick, I've been reading and I think that your fractured orbit is causing a pinched nerve. Paint one lens of your glasses with clear nail-polish and when it is nearly dry, smear it. Then your eye can get light, not the darkness behind the patch.' So much love, so much concern and usually an explanation or suggestion that was really useful. For the first five years, this nail-polished lens was the most useful thing I found to deal with the double vision. All the visits to all those specialists, and nothing helped me as much as Dad's suggestion!

My family continued to be saintly and would only occasionally slip out a 'You told us that only a second ago'. Ann, Helen and Ken shopped, cooked, cleaned, drove me to countless doctor and hospital appointments and patiently waited with me. They sat with me, tried to cheer me up when I was low and always had fresh coffee for my visitors. Rob was particularly good at patting me when I wept. Ted hovered around us all, trying to think of anything to alleviate my pain and boredom. He had been married to someone who was always interested, busy, happy and full of wonder at the world, now his wife was a lifeless being who felt no pleasure in anything.

My passion for life had totally melted away. I felt flat and one-dimensional, not the full and multi-dimensional person I had been. I was not a patient patient. Lurking in a hidden part of my brain fluttered the thought 'When I am better, will I get better? Will I *ever* be better? Will I *ever* be the 'old' me?'

The 'old' me loved reading, water-colour painting, music, playing piano, piano accordion and guitar, going to concerts, plays and films, visiting galleries, browsing around the shops with friends or daughters, eating out, entertaining, often with 20 people for a breakfast in the sun on the deck. The country was another passion of the 'old' me: bushwalking, riding the old motorbike, horse and donkey-riding, and mucking around at the family country weekender. I remembered standing around a campfire on a school camping trip, squeezing my old piano accordion as the kids' voices leapt to the tall gum trees with the bright sparks of the fire. But the fire had gone out of this 'new' me.

My mother had always said to the 'old' me 'You are not a human be-ing, you are a human do-er!' My happiness/satisfaction/contentment/peace came as a result of 'doing'. 'Doing' gave me a sense of achievement. I always had lists and plans for things to do in the future. The children would joke they'd put 'She always had a rake or broom in her hand' on my tombstone. It had always felt so good when I had everything neat and tidy, proof (to myself) that I was in control of my world. I'd loved nothing better than getting stuck into the half-acre of garden, mowing and planting. When our swimming pool was installed I had carried two tons of pavers the 150 feet down the hill from the road in a few days; numerous trips carrying two pavers wrapped in an old T-shirt! This 'new' me was incapable of carrying a cup without breaking it!

Travel, especially off the beaten track, had really turned on the 'old' me: What could be more exciting than exploring Portuguese Timor in a truck, walking through the rice paddies of Bali, or pottering about the back streets of Indonesia in the freshness of dawn with the moon still hovering in the pink sky? Having travelled extensively as a child through Africa, Europe and India the travel bug was well entrenched. A trip to Europe with the four kids to give them a white Christmas had been a highlight of our lives. This 'new' me shook with fear just to be driven to the local shops.

In retrospect, 'faulty thinking' was a dark place in the labyrinth

I used to believe the way I saw things was the truth. Years later, when I learnt about faulty thinking, I suddenly saw I'd become an expert faulty thinker: I filtered things so that I only saw things as good or bad; I saw things as either black or white and I couldn't see the grey area in between. I generally over-generalised and jumped to conclusions. I became skilled at catastrophising. I always took things personally and believed things should be 'fair' as I saw it. My faulty thinking led to so much unhappiness.

In retrospect, blaming myself was a dark place in the labyrinth

For a long time I told myself, 'If only you'd done such and such you might have improved more!' 'Why didn't you do...!' But then I remembered Ivy's story. Her husband had a severe stroke and for many years she'd nursed and helped him, often being perplexed by the crazy things this once brilliant man did: he set fire to the curtains, ran away from home and attacked her with a poker.

One afternoon Dick went missing for several hours. She searched everywhere until she eventually found him, down the back garden, sitting in the disused outside toilet. He had a rubbish bin on his knees and 15 neckties around his neck. She managed to drag the bin off his knees and pull him out of the small outhouse. Then she took him by the shoulders and said 'Why did you do it Dick? Why?' She did not expect a rational explanation and was astounded when he said *'Because at the time it seemed like a good idea'*.

When I look back on how I've tried to recapture my life I can repeat Dick's words — at the time it seemed a good idea, the right thing to do. I've never said to myself 'I'm going to do this because it is a stupid idea'. Every step of the way I've tried to do the right thing so I should stop blaming myself.

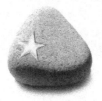

11.
Getaway to the coast

The trip was like a nightmare. The road to Lorne was so dangerous.
At first the thought of how long we'd be trapped in the car
When we'd had 'the' accident filled my brain.
Then as we got closer to Lorne the thought
Of the trip in the ambulance scared me witless.
Tomorrow we have to drive home.

Ted suggested a short getaway to the seaside town of Lorne. He believed I'd be a different person with two nights away from home. Wow! I really needed to be a different person but there was so much fear to conquer to leave home. Just getting into the car was a challenge. I'd been told in rehab that the chances of being involved in a second accident were slim, but so were the odds of having the first accident and that had happened!

So with my heart in my mouth we drove first to Queenscliff, two hours away. Sitting beside a roaring fire in a room full to overflowing with luscious bowls of flowers I felt the nightmare shimmer and shift. The pain was still as ghastly, and I flopped in our room for my afternoon nap, but I started to believe that perhaps I might be a 'real' person again.

Before dinner we took a stroll along the pier and around the town. Even though I had to feel the way, touching trees, fences and railings to get my bearings, I could sense the calm and beauty of the evening. Dinner was superb and I only knocked my knife off the table once and spilt only a little food. Things were indeed looking up. We had a cheery fire glowing in our room when we went upstairs and I felt the shadow of happiness flowing in my veins for the first time in months.

Unfortunately and unbelievably, I awoke at midnight shaking with pain and the most violent gastric attack I'd ever suffered, and ended up spending the night in the quaint bathroom across the hall. Weeks and tests later confirmed that I'd picked up a nasty bug in hospital. Why did it choose that night to rear its ugly head? After a squeamish breakfast in the delightful breakfast room came another big decision: to stay another night in Queenscliff or drive on to Lorne. My inclination was to stay another night, but Ted had a passion to go further down the coast.

Somehow I managed to endure the winding road to Lorne along the Great Ocean Road. Ted helped me into the room, and then sat me on the patio with the view of the sea and coastline stretching out in front of us. He then left me and went into the township. When he'd gone, I cried my eyes out. Was my howling just a reaction to the dangerous drive? Was it the double waving horizon line making me sick? Was it a longing to be as I was this time last year, when we'd bounded down to town for a coffee, full of happiness? In anger and frustration I left the patio and threw myself down on the motel bed, badly miscalculating distance and banging my head violently on the bed-head. When I opened my eyes I was bitterly disappointed. I still couldn't see properly!

Ted returned, proudly sporting ten red tulips in a borrowed vase. Five months earlier, when we had been in New York, Ted had bought me ten pink tulips and put them in a milk carton. When I thought about it, it was the same sentiment, same flowers, same number, same Ted, *but* a different country, different colours, a different container and a *different me*. Weeping, I removed the eye-patch and there were twice as many flowers, twice the sentiment and twice the gratitude.

Ted said he'd give his right arm or ten years of his life to take away my pain. Just knowing of the offer made the pain more bearable. It's strange that for four months we'd been unable to discuss how we really felt about the accident. I had felt Ted's anger and now, years later, can recognise it for what it was — anger at the man who did this to me, the person who had changed our lives. At the time I felt so different, ungainly, out of control, stupid and unlovable, I secretly thought he must be angry at me for wrecking our lives.

Sitting at a table in the fish and chip shop, biting into a piece of flake, Ted said he was so glad to see a shine back in my (unpatched) eye. He spoke of sad nights at dinner when my lifeless eye nearly broke his heart. He said he loved me. How could he? I felt so completely unlovable. He became angry when I wept. I tried to explain how I felt and he then explained that he was upset and frustrated that he could not help me. We had been married for 25 years and had always shared our hopes and beliefs and fears. But without any experience of this situation, and with no counselling, how were we to know how to tackle things? Ted somehow blamed himself that I had had the accident, as if it was his task in life to protect me and he had failed. He wanted to fix the problems; perhaps another specialist, more cushions or a painkiller could stop my tears. We then realised that all our energies were directed at trying to make life seem normal as quickly as possible for the kids. We were playing a game that life was still the same. Now we had both the time and inclination to start bringing out some of our fears and hopes into the open.

Taxi-drivers who did the rehab run would tell me that the saddest part about accidents was how they break up marriages, or as one driver put it, 'The tiniest hairline crack would widen and split them apart'. I suppose our trip to Lorne was like super-glue.

When we returned home I wrote:

'I think I'm starting to feel a little better. Today I saw two little girls, Brownies, sitting on a wall. There was a woman peeping through the blinds at the sight of her new front fence. I could feel her glee and happiness. A black dog with white socks was trotting through the gate after his master — faithfulness and warm fur — wonderful animals. It's funny that I haven't seen scenes like this for months.'

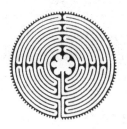

12.

University: Trying to find 'Me' and get out of the labyrinth

I've discovered that we only see what we look at.
I've discovered that it's hard to know where to look.
I've discovered that it's hard to understand what you see.

I had a one-track mind. I decided that if I could get back to university and work on my Master's degree, I would find the 'old' me. I just had to try and do it. After much soul-searching and working-out of practicalities such as who would drive and pick me up we decided that I should try to continue my study. In a way it felt like my pain and suffering would all have been in vain if I gave up. Somehow, to continue my education seemed a positive active step in preventing Mr X from ruining my life.

In hindsight my first night of lectures alone was crazy! The trip in to uni terrified me. Ted drove me there, helped find the lecture room, sat me in a seat and, bless his heart, stayed and took notes for me. Ken, Helen and Ann each volunteered to accompany and help me.

Because the subject was a sequel to one I'd completed in a summer school at the beginning of the year, just before the

...ontent and much of the terminology were familiar. ...ekly two-hour evening lecture. Rick, the lecturer, ...ortive and helpful and my fellow students were ...er, it felt as if everyone was speaking a foreign ...nguage and I could not understand a word. Fortunately Rick ran the classes by giving notes to read at home before the lecture.

At home the kids read the notes to me. Still they made no sense. After several weeks of perseverance and discussions with Ken and Helen about the topic, I started to understand a little. Ted increased the size of the type of the notes, and I used a ruler and finger to slowly follow each line and repeated them out loud. Gradually, I understood fragments of what Rick was talking about. How excited I felt when I could grasp the meaning of a sentence! This was working. By putting in a tremendous effort I could improve. Slowly, slowly I could try to recapture this section of my life.

In the past I'd typed my projects on a typewriter but the boys felt a computer would help. It did. The computer meant that I could slowly make notes in big print. It became possible for ideas to come out via my one 'typing finger' on the keyboard when it would have been hard to say or read the words.

It was so interesting. I could not understand a novel but to study a familiar subject was possible, with heaps of help and encouragement from my family. At times I would record ideas on a tape as I lay in bed and the kids would type them up. Study certainly provided an activity I could do at my own pace when I felt well enough. Even if it was just ten minutes a day I felt as if I was achieving something. If I had time to spend waiting for an appointment with the physio or the doctor, I'd pull out a page or two of notes and a marker.

Tutorials were another thing altogether. They were a huge challenge because I had such trouble speaking and reading out loud and my memory was so poor. I could read the same paragraph over and over again and not realise I'd just read it. Placing my finger on each word helped, but was rather slow and ungainly for presenting a uni paper. So I found things that could become cues and help me to speak. I thought of using several different boxes or chests with matches or chess pieces in them to help me get the message across. Pictures and symbols and charts written by Ann spoke to me and my audience. Of course, this meant that Ken or Ann had to get me and my bag of tricks to and from uni.

Uni was a wonderful measure by which to gauge my progress. We graduated from Ted having to take me by the hand, physically put me in a chair and put a pencil in my hand, to Ken supporting my weight as we fumbled our way to the lecture, and then to Ann just leading me across the road. Then came the day when she waited and watched in the car, heart in her mouth, while I crossed the road on my own at the pedestrian crossing. Later she said she felt just as I must have as I watched her learn to cross the road at primary school. Talk about role reversal!

Nowadays I was the one to make the house untidy and the kids had to pick up after me. Ann would still put out my clothes because I didn't know what kind of clothes I liked or what shirt went with what pants or jacket. Ann was a great help to me when it came to getting dressed. She seemed to forever be saying: 'Oh Mum you can't go out looking like that! Come here and I will do up your buttons in the right holes!'

Another role reversal happened when Ann took me to a large shopping complex to help me move about among people and I saw someone eating a pie. I decided I wanted one for lunch. It had been years since I'd tried to eat a pie out of a paper bag. Immediately, I was covered in pie and I couldn't even begin to figure out what to do, so I just went on trying to eat the pie. It didn't occur to me to try to wipe up the mess. Ann disappeared, I panicked. I couldn't blame her for running away from me because she was ashamed of me — I'd run away from me if I could. I was ashamed of me too! So I stood there in the busy forecourt dripping with pie and tears. I didn't know my name, I didn't know where I lived, I didn't know how I'd get home. Ann reappeared clutching a handful of paper serviettes and carefully cleaned me up and led me to the car.

The episode of the pie unsettled me. I told myself I was crazy to be so upset about this when dreadful things were happening in the world. People were dying in wars, children were starving and I was so shallow to be upset by a bit of pie. But that pie was a symbol that I, mother of four, teacher of 500, wiper-up extraordinaire of messes, foreseer of potential messes was totally lost and powerless.

 In retrospect, just because something seems small it doesn't meant it can't have big ramifications

Back then I often said to myself 'Don't be so upset. It's silly to cry about spilt milk or broken plates or falling over in public. They're only small things compared to the terrible things that are happening to other people.'

Then one day my physio told me a story that helped me make sense of feeling foolish. He'd often tell me stories to try to distract me from my pain, and this day he spoke about his passion for yacht racing, and how he nearly perished the previous weekend. He'd won his first yacht race with flying colours, and although the weather, crew and yacht were the same for the second race he'd replaced the lynch pin between races and forgotten to bend it. It fell out and was lost overboard, the tiller became useless, they could not steer the boat and the crew ended up in the ocean. A slight bend of the pin was such a small part of the entire sailing experience, yet it was so important and its loss nearly had devastating consequences.

This story brought home to me how small things can have big ramifications; how small changes to our lives can have devastating consequences. Even the tiniest changes can become symbols of how our life is not the same anymore.

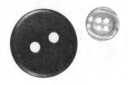

13.
School: Trying to find 'Me' and get out of the labyrinth

I've discovered that doing something useful helps you feel good about yourself.
I've discovered that my concept of who I am is tied up with what I do.
I've discovered that the more you try to forget something the more you will remember.
I've discovered that the more you try to remember something the more you will forget.

I had an overwhelming wish to return to teaching. 'How could you possibly teach?' I hear you ask. That I even contemplated such a thing is an example of how muddled my thinking was. I was still experiencing horrific pain with my ribs poking out like a bird's wing in my back. My left leg dragged, and this brought on unbelievable muscle pain. Frequently I could not walk when I first woke up, and I would have to crawl upstairs to the rest of the house in the morning. My left hand was clenched, my palm constantly marked by my nails.

I was suffering from fatigue, so I only had a couple of good hours a day. I had double vision, I had times when I blacked out momentarily, and all in all I was still in a very bad way. Mentally

I felt completely hopeless. I couldn't understand or remember things. My sense of time, space and numbers had gone. Yet, I insisted that I would get back to school! It really was too early in my recovery, but I was adamant.

School meant so much to me: the students, my colleagues, the ideas. It was my life. I just couldn't imagine life without teaching. In order to recapture my old life I felt I had to return to school. Every day since I left hospital I'd thought, 'When I get back to school, life will be right again'.

Fran, the understanding person from rehab, was there to assist me to find my way back to work. She was there to protect me from failing, to be supportive and pick up the pieces when the going got tough. It was her task to analyse the job requirements and to try to match my skills to the job. She also had to make sure I was not a danger to myself or others. She had to explain to the Head of the school that people who suffered from acquired brain damage may display fatigue, difficulty in concentration and loss of memory. She did not list all my deficits as she felt that doing so would only make them more obvious.

No-one knew what progress I would make. It was apparent that not one of the specialists believed that I would be able to return to full-time teaching. Of course this was just like a red rag to a bull, and made me even more determined to prove them all wrong. Notwithstanding every ounce of effort I have put into getting better, I must now admit they were right, but I wasn't to know this at the time. Indeed, if I had known that five years later, I would only be able to work two mornings a week, I might have given up completely and wallowed in despair.

After many lengthy discussions between the school, the doctors, the hospital and Fran, it was decided that I was not yet ready to return to my Grade Six girls. I was absolutely shattered. I had tried so hard to get better and I'd failed. I felt I'd not only failed myself, but also my family and my school and last, but not least, my pupils and their families. My pupils had kept regular contact with me in the expectation I would return to be their teacher in the fourth term. I tried to explain the situation to them by writing a letter to each of them, to go with a made-up 'Rehab Report'.

Rehabilitation Report on Chris Durham

1. WALKING — BALANCE — EYESIGHT

Chris is learning to scan where she is going before she walks through doorways. This skill is reducing damage both to door frames and her arms. She is trying hard with her balance exercises and is of less danger to herself and others.

She is learning to monitor herself when she feels she is 'floating'. As she still has a lot of trouble judging distance and depth, we recommend she takes out a new insurance policy to cover breakages.

Chris should make sure there isn't a car in sight when she steps out on to the road, even though she is learning new vocabulary from people driving the cars she walks in front of.

When pouring a cup of coffee, a finger in the mug to judge depth will save wiping up spills.

2. TALKING

Chris is finding ways of coping when she a) forgets words; b) makes up strange words; c) forgets what she is talking about; and d) forgets what you are talking about.

3. SHOPPING

Chris must take greater care not to queue-jump through not scanning properly, as this tends to cause awkward moments. She must also take more care when walking near large stacks of cans — this can cause even more difficult moments.

4. OTHER
More work still needs to be put into doing up buttons, not dropping things or knocking over vases, people or cups, or stepping on dogs or cats.
5. HOMEWORK
Chris must learn to slow down and rest for ten minutes each hour.

How could I explain to kids about double vision? I wrote 'Chris's Song', to be sung to the last verse of 'The twelve days of Christmas'.

> *'When I get up each morning this is what I see...two right hands, two cheery husbands, two black dogs, two cakes of soap...two shiny toasters...two bowls of flowers, two Helens, two Kens, two Anns and two tall Robs. And then I put my eye-patch on!'*

It was decided that I would return to school for a couple of mornings a week to do alternative duties. I was to be a 'useful person', listing equipment in the science and maths store rooms, helping in the library, covering books and so on. After several weeks of this regime I was to take a half-hour philosophy and discussion session as enrichment or extension with a group of five girls. After a couple more weeks I would take two small group classes, widely interspersed with my library work.

I must confess my first morning at school was a bit of a disaster. For a start the kids all wanted to hug me, which was a trifle painful, but it was wonderful to be with the kids and my colleagues, to catch up on their news, and to feel part of the school again. But there was the strange sensation of not belonging, of not having a spot to call my own. Although I still had a passionate interest in the kids from my grade, they were no longer 'mine'. In fairness to them and their new teacher, I had to let them go.

I started cataloguing the science equipment, weeping silently into my eye-patch. Let me tell you, a soggy eye-patch is no fun. I badly wanted to be useful, but it took so long for me to understand or do things. Tasks that before would have been done in a flash now required amazing concentration, not only to grasp what the task was, but to remember what I was doing. I seemed to have incredible difficulty with concepts, ideas and even remembering why I was at school but not in my classroom. I was constantly having to remember 'I've had an accident, that's why I'm doing this'.

The library was my salvation — a bottomless pit of new books to process and labels to stick. The concentration required was perfect rehab: teaching my hands to obey me, relearning the alphabet, learning to work with the double vision. I was very fortunate that the school supported me as they did even though they had a great deal of concern about what sort of legal liability I would present were I to fall!

After several weeks I started working with one group, then two groups of five girls, for half an hour each morning, holding philosophy/thinking discussions. This was both wonderful and terrible. I had great difficulty planning the half-hour sessions, so I used work that I'd written up before the accident. What amazing discussions we had, but how frustrating as well! No matter what I did I couldn't remember students' names or what we were talking about a minute after we'd discussed something. Was this progress? It was exciting to be a 'teacher' again, but somehow I knew I was not the same teacher I had been.

As the year drew to a close, my hopes that I would reclaim the 'old' me faded. As my pain improved, but as I attempted to do more, I gained a greater understanding of my problems.

When I was not taking philosophy/thinking sessions I continued my struggle with helping in the library. The students were magnificent. I've never had any discipline problems, apart from the students getting a little loud in their enthusiasm; they were kind, tolerant, friendly, interested and understanding. I contribute much of my satisfaction and happiness to the wonderful support of the girls.

In order to follow our discussions I would make notes on a large sheet of paper. My spelling had gone the same way as my maths. The students kindly helped me by correcting my work. I had quite a bit of trouble writing as I had forgotten the alphabet, and would put unrelated letters in words. In the older groups one student or another would say, 'Don't worry, Mrs D, we'll write for you'. It's most humbling to have a student take the marker pen from your fingers to take over the role of recorder.

The new Prep students would think I was a pirate lady or that I had no eye beneath the patch, but once I had shown them my eye they accepted it, and only occasionally needed to check — just to make certain it was still there. I hope I didn't cause them nightmares about a one-eyed lady!

Helen and Ann started a collection of walking sticks with different heads. The students loved to open one stick which has a compass and flask; they patted the duck head or horse's head that formed the handle on the other sticks. Sometimes I would come across a group of girls 'playing philosophy', having very meaningful conversations, where the leader had a blackboard ruler as a walking stick, and my stick seemed to be constantly in demand as a prop for plays; so much so that I kept a spare stick at school to lend to the girls who needed it.

Over the next few years remembering my students' names challenged and frustrated me. I first made cardboard name labels to place in front of each student. This was a dismal failure as they all tended to play with them, or, worse still, bang them on the table which was trying to my double vision and sensitive hearing. Then I prepared name labels with a loop of different coloured ribbon to place around a top button on their school uniform. This also failed as it took too long to give them out. Next I asked them to bring a plastic name tag from home — also not a good idea as they often forgot to bring the name tag. I tried getting them to write their names on the page they were working on, but this didn't solve my problem as they often forgot. Yet I took this trouble because I realised that if people do not know, or forget our name, we can think they do not like or value us. It took me two years of frustration, shame and anger before I came up with a solution to my name problem. Not string but wool.

I developed a lesson where wool became a concrete example of the way philosophy/thinking sessions would progress. Not the usual back and forth between students and teacher, which is like the spokes of a fan. Instead I would hold the end of a ball of wool and throw the ball across the table to a student who'd hold a section it and then throw the ball to another student, who'd repeat the process. We would end up with a rather strange looking spider's web. I'd ask the class how a spider uses a web. 'To trap food' would be the reply. Then I'd explain that I forgot things, and how sometimes we all had difficulty remembering things; and needed something that could a trap for our thoughts — a 'thinking trap'. So our philosophy journals would be called 'Thinking Traps'.

After starting a discussion I would throw the messy ball of wool to someone to start the conversation — they got the ball rolling. After they'd made their point they'd throw the ball of wool to someone who wanted to add to the discussion. When they held the wool they had the floor. Names were no longer crucial and the students could run the discussions amongst themselves. Holding, pulling, winding and unwinding the wool had a most amazing spin-off; it seemed to loosen tongues and thoughts. It was also a non-threatening way to stop certain students from hogging the discussion. It was much easier to say, 'You've had the wool several times' than 'You talk all the time'. A couple of times a lesson I'd ask them to pass the wool around so that everyone, even the very shy, contributed to the discussion.

I must confess this wool business led to some quite crazy episodes, like the time several girls were 'busting' with ideas only to be told in a superior way by the person speaking 'I've got the wool so listen to me!' It was quite a spectacle. Not to be beaten, the frustrated 'speaker-to-be' spied a scrap of red wool on a shelf (we shared our room with Craft) and held it aloft saying 'I've got the wool!' The holder of the ball of wool quickly retorted, 'No! It's got to be a *ball* of red wool!' At lightning speed the other student rubbed her hands together, rolling the scrap into a minute ball which she displayed to us between her fingertips. As you can imagine by this time we were all rolling round the floor laughing, but we quietened down enough for her to put forward her point.

Because I couldn't follow a written curriculum, I devised ways to use objects to stimulate the kids' interest and curiosity. Giving each student a five cent piece, we would describe and discuss cents, scents and sense. Another session was based on baked beans. I placed a can of baked beans on the table and said 'Our lesson is in the can'. The students were full of curiosity. We discussed beans, and I asked what story had beans in it. 'Jack and the Beanstalk,' was the reply. We then debated whether Jack was good or bad, giving reasons for the positions. I was astounded to hear some five year olds ask 'Was Jack good, to kill the bad giant?' 'Is it bad to kill a good person?' 'How do we know if someone is good or bad?'

After I'd finished a morning teaching it felt strange to be standing at the school gate at noon, waiting for the taxi that would take me home. On arriving home I would fall into bed and sleep soundly for several hours, frequently waking so deathly cold it was frightening. Somehow I'd manage to stiffly struggle to the shower and stand under near boiling water for up to 20 minutes, but I would still feel frozen to the bone. My brain injury meant that my body didn't control my temperature correctly.

Then it would be time to psych myself up to appear normal when the family arrived home. What a life! What a waste of a life!

During this time I'd been patchless for a couple of months. Then I was told by the same specialist to put my patch back on. The complexity of my double vision was starting to emerge as my eyes settled down. Apparently both eyes were twisted from the horizontal and vertical planes. I did not see the ground as level with either eye. I had hoped surgery could straighten up one eye to the other, but according to the specialist, both eyes had to be moved. Several operations to each eye were discussed. There was also a likelihood that the eyes would revert to how they were despite the surgery. My eye-surgeon referred me to yet another specialist but he was not keen to operate yet. More time was needed for my eyes to settle.

I was absolutely devastated. My plans of returning to school to take Grade Six the following year were dashed. The bitterest blow of the year was accepting the advice of the medicos that I would not be fit for full-time duties for some time.

Thinking back on it all, I can remember my dogged determination that 'I will teach next year', despite all the evidence to hand indicating that I would not be able to cope. I can't describe the sadness and despair I felt as Ted helped me remove all my gear from my classroom. Would I ever have my own class again? Would I ever use all my charts and pictures and books again? I wept as we placed all my stuff in boxes and Ted carted them to the school attic. I just hoped that soon, I would need them again.

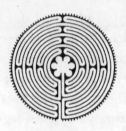

14.
Reality and unreality clash

In the blink of an eye
I am in that surreal other world
That strange world
The 7th dimension, virtual reality
Where unreality is more real than reality.

As 1991 drew to a close, six months after the accident, I started to find myself on the most amazing, surreal trips. I would be doing something like biting into a cherry, when suddenly I would find myself a 12-year-old, sitting in a tree with my brother. These frequent 'trips' were more vivid than reality, brighter than technicolour. They were like the nightmares I had experienced in hospital. I'd detect a pungent burning smell and check the stove and the iron to see if I'd inadvertently left them on. It was too difficult to explain to anyone, too weird. It was my terrible secret — I was mad.

On one of my numerous visits to the neurologist she remarked that I had damage to the area of my brain that epileptics have damaged. She asked me if I was having epileptic fits. 'Oh no,' I answered with surety. I'd had teacher training. I knew that an epileptic fit was when you lay on the floor and needed a ruler

Reality and unreality clash

between your teeth. I didn't think to report that when I first came round in intensive care I discovered I'd bitten a large chunk of my tongue off. I think I did mention how it drove me crazy that I was frequently nipping my tongue with my teeth. This hurt so much it would constantly wake me up.

Early in the New Year these issues came up once more. Again I tried to voice my blanking-out episodes. This time I received an explanation for my trips: epilepsy. I wasn't going mad. Relief washed over me.

I was prescribed Tegretol. The effects of the drug were wonderful. It seemed to unlock part of my brain so that I could think with greater clarity, make connections and links. Somehow messages seemed to get through. I felt almost normal. Three weeks later though, I felt really odd.

One Sunday morning Ted took me to the doctor. 'I don't know what's wrong but my whole body feels out of control...I'm scared...could I be having a reaction to the drugs?' Unfortunately Hugh wasn't on that morning and the doctor and I got sidetracked discussing chest infections and other things. (Chest infections hovered about me constantly, and I subsequently learnt from specialists in New York that this is common with head injury.)

Antibiotics were prescribed. Despite taking them, in the following days I had to return to the doctor. The antibiotics were changed. A week passed. I lay in my glass room, moaning. I became sicker and sicker, my heart felt as if it was squashed by an elephant, I had a fever and terrible pains in my joints and I could only walk a couple of steps at a time. Another week went by and tests indicated possible hepatitis and heart troubles. We waited days to find out what sort of hepatitis it was. Throughout this trauma, my only aim in life was to eat a potato so that I wouldn't take my epilepsy drugs on an empty stomach. I writhed on my bed. I was sure I was dying. When I started to vomit up white soapy stuff, my mind flashed to the story of Madame Bovary and how she died after taking poison. 'I'm being poisoned', I told myself. And indeed I was — I discussed it with Hugh and he agreed it could be strong reaction to the epilepsy drug. The only way to be sure was to stop taking it.

Slowly I recovered, although my heart and liver were damaged. Rather than try another drug it seemed safer to try to manage the epilepsy without medication. After a couple of years the seizures became less frequent. Initially I had several a day, and now I may experience only one blanking-out a week.

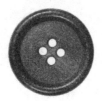

15.
End of the year my life changed

I've planted punnet after punnet of seedlings.
For me they're a talisman, a symbol
That come Christmas they'll flower into a facsimile of the flower on the label,
And I hope that come Christmas I'll flower too
That I'll flower into my old self.

I was still experiencing difficulty trying to appear normal. The way I walked and talked made me appear as if I was a little drunk all the time. I certainly had to learn to be less sensitive about the way people would take a step back and watch my ungainly gait as I tried to feel my way about. I felt very much a 'lesser person' when people would retreat from me, as I struggled to find the post and the pedestrian lights on my way to an appointment in the city.

Care and concentration were needed trying to cross the road and the railway line near school. One morning I ran in front of an oncoming train. I saw the safety barrier go down and didn't remember what it signified. I did remember being a child in a running race and the finishing line ribbon. I confused the two objects and ran across the train tracks with my stick and bag of school books.

I had to try to remember to only cross the road at traffic lights.

With visual inattention and my poor visuo-spatial ability, I'd become lost in supermarkets, school and at home. Getting lost and mis-seeing things left me feeling confused and frightened, upset and stupid.

Tears of frustration and sadness would spring out of my eyes when I forgot words, or didn't understand the meanings of words — there had been little improvement in my comprehension. My coping strategy was to pretend that I understood what was going on or what people said. At school, my day-to-day comprehension difficulties and forgetfulness made conversations with staff gruelling, most of the time I was confused and bewildered. I was unable to initiate an important conversation without first making notes. Often I was full of overwhelming dread and fear as I couldn't grasp what was going on. This exacerbated my anxiety, and led to me wanting to withdraw from social contact.

It felt so silly to have to make notes to have a discussion with Ted. I must also have been an incredibly irritating person to have a discussion with, because I had to say what I wanted to say when I thought of it, or else I'd lose the thought. This meant I had to interrupt people when they were speaking or make notes. After some time I realised that I needed to know the topic people were talking about before I could understand what they were saying or make links in my head. Ted might be in full flight telling me about something, and I'd need to stop him and ask him to explain how his comments fitted into the discussion.

I was also plagued by a lack of common-sense and judgment. My frontal-lobe damage meant it was difficult to control emotions and behave appropriately. I later learnt that this was the reason I was too familiar with strangers and frequently said inappropriate and confronting things.

As the end of the year approached, changes were afoot. Helen obtained vacation work in Thailand, so she went off for four months to work in a large law firm in Bangkok. We had gone to live in Thailand when she was in Grade Six. All the kids but Rob had attended the International School there. Rob had clung to my knees as I studied for a Bachelor of Education by correspondence at home in the comparative cool of the mornings. The kids would arrive home at lunchtime, school over for the day, and we would spend the afternoons together. Weekends would be spent exploring the city and the culture, or at the British Club. We'd all loved the sights, sounds and smells of Asia.

Helen's boyfriend, Greg, went to Thailand to join her and they returned home happy and engaged. We were all thrilled. Greg had been so much a part of the family for several years. A musician, his song, written to wish Helen a happy birthday on her 21st birthday, became a big hit.

Helen's move to Thailand allowed Ann to move into Helen's room in a student house. Suddenly I'd lost two of my supporters. Life was not going to be as pleasant. I could not help but feel that Ann must have been secretly relieved to leave home. I was glad she would have some freedom, but sad to lose her company and help. She would still come home to cook, shop and clean up, but I felt lost without my 'live-in' companion. I was now completely dependent on the boys: Ken was continuing with his Arts degree and Rob was in Year Eleven at school.

The year my life changed was drawing to a close. Christmas morning we woke up to the sound of carols floating up the valley from the park, where the local band play an annual dawn concert. I reflected on how wonderful the family had been. Later in the day as I rested in the glass-room, I tried to find a way of expressing how I felt as the year ended. The flutter of a bird's wing caught my eye. That's it, I thought! The story of the birds and my one 'late bloomer' tells it all.

> 'I think it was early summer when the magpies made their first appearance for the year. There was a mum, dad and four babies. From my bed in the glass-room overlooking the valley I watched with interest as this family paid a visit to the bird feeding-tray in a nearby tree. My slow and painful recovery had been cheered by the daily visits of my many feathered friends.

The seasons passed and the birds changed with them. The curlews, the wild doves that cooed as they ruffled their pinkish breasts, the four kookaburras who waiting expectantly until I scrounged some meat for them, and now the faithful magpies, had returned for yet another season of singing for their supper, and delighting us with their antics to repay us for providing them with a restaurant.

From the first day my eye was caught by one of the babies. This bird was smaller than the other babies and it perched in the tree, watching as its greedy siblings were fed by the parents. It made twice the noise of the others, but frequently appeared to miss out entirely on being fed because it was so busy squawking. Weeks and months passed till the babies were as large as their parents but still would clamour to be fed by their poor parents (I suppose our kids are as tall, if not taller than us and they still need us to provide the food!).

By this time I felt quite worried about my 'slow one', as I'd called him. I'd noticed that, like me, he had great trouble balancing to walk; he stumbled, and at times missed the branch or feeding-tray when he landed. I tried putting out two lots of food, hoping he would be able to feed in peace, but the others would quickly tackle the new pile of food. I was sure that the scrawny, noisy bird would perish.

But then, this skinny, lone magpie would come at odd times, calling to have the food in the tray replenished; when he was with his family he started to pick up the oats they had spilt during their feeding frenzy.

Then one day as I went to the laundry door there was a plump, sleek magpie sifting through the scraps in the compost bucket. My 'slow one' was the only one from the magpie family to realise that just around the corner was a constant supply of food. He is still a little clumsy at times and hangs back from the crowd, but he has found his own way of coping and getting by.'

My magpie showed me that in order to thrive, I needed to find alternative ways, to look in different places. I'd be better off to look to the back door of life to give me opportunities.

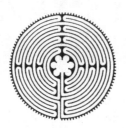

16.
Caught in court — a labyrinth within a labyrinth

Dancing with the lawyer for the Defence.
I was put in an excruciating position today.
I could think and feel outrage for the way you were 'playing' with my emotions
Deep inside my head warning bells were ringing
I knew you were trying to trap me yet I could not process or comprehend
I certainly could not follow your dance step
As you kept changing the tune.

One Saturday morning Ted took me to the police station to make a statement. The young police officer remembered me and gave me time to try to put together my statement. He spoke of holding the intravenous drip for me as I was being attended by the ambulance crew. He said how he felt frustrated with the man who had hit me because he appeared so indifferent and uncaring. In chatting after we had completed the paperwork, he said his sister had gone to Ivanhoe Girls' Grammar and when he repeated his surname I realised I had taught her. It's a small world.

In the New Year I was subpoenaed to be a witness in the

Criminal Court. I was still in considerable pain, I had difficulty walking and my thinking and reasoning were slow and laborious which meant that I had difficulty grasping the meanings of conversations, and speaking was a huge effort. We called in to meet the police officer contesting the case; he told me to relax and just tell the truth. The police had charged Mr X with dangerous driving, failing to stop at a stop sign and failing to render assistance.

I was to appear as a witness on the first day of court. Ted and I sat outside the courtroom, waiting. It was a thrill to see Peter, who had saved my life, but I felt so guilty that he had to miss work because of my court case. A stranger came up and introduced himself to me, and so I learnt of how Steve, a passing tow-truck driver, had helped Peter to smash the passenger-side window to break into the car and take off the seat-belt that was choking me. Steve was pleased to see me alive. It felt strange to be in the court waiting room with a stranger kneeling before me, holding my hands. We beamed at each other.

Another man was sitting on another bench. That had to be the dreaded Mr X. I looked at him and for a few seconds felt nothing. Then I was overwhelmed with waves of fury, confusion and pain.

I was called into court. The door opened and I was swallowed up in a room with no windows. I was overcome by claustrophobia. Panic surfaced. All I could think was that I was only a few seats from the man who had ruined my life. I wanted to scream and shout, to point at him and say, 'Look what you've done!'

The police had done a trade-off with the other side; they would drop the 'failing to stop at a stop sign' charge if the lawyer from the other side would be 'gentle with me'. However, I still had to remain silent and listen to his lawyer explain that it was all *my* fault. You could have knocked me over with a feather when this line of assertion finally managed to filter through into my mind.

Once I took the stand his lawyer asked me if I would be too

upset to look at a photo of the street where the accident occurred. My mind did a backflip. What? It was not *the road* that nearly killed, me it was *that man*! My mind was in a furious whirlwind.

He showed me a photo of the accident site with large trucks parked along the road. 'He only poked the front of his car out to see past the trucks.'

I couldn't understand. The day I had the accident there were no trucks there (later we checked and the road was a no parking zone). The world had gone mad. The way things had happened had all seemed so obvious, so simple, that I just couldn't believe my ears and mind. I could hardly follow the crazy ideas that were being put forward. Then it was suggested I was speeding, because I was in a hurry.

From the recesses of my mind floated the fact that I was early that day and had no reason to hurry. I can't remember if the right words came out of my mouth.

The pain in my back felt like a chainsaw. The world was whirling round me. I could only manage two hours in court that day. Ted took me home during the lunch break, put me to bed, and then he returned for the rest of the sitting.

There were another two days of court but there was no way I could have attended or coped with it. Ted and my parents attended each sitting, which were spread out over the period of a month. Ted would return home after each day in court to inform me of the proceedings. Of how Mr X would say how he smashed the window to turn off the ignition, and Peter would explain that no, the driver's window had been down so he just had to put his hand through the open window. It became a battle between Mr X and Peter. Apparently Peter was a superb witness (according to the police, the best witness they'd ever had). At last Mr X was found guilty of dangerous driving and failing to render assistance. His punishment was a fine of one thousand dollars and two years off the road.

I was surprised to find that having my day in court helped me accept and come to terms with having the accident. It was almost as if the hearing was an acknowledgment of the event. The accident *had* occurred. My life *had* changed. It was good to let go and stop focusing on Mr X, and to try to get on with the rest of our lives.

The next episode came from our insurance company. Mr X claimed that I was partly responsible for the accident — so once again we went onto the court merry-go-round.

At this time I was very ill — a reaction to the anti-epilepsy drug. I could not eat, I shook, my heart felt as if it was tearing out of my body, I could hardly walk and yet I had to somehow go to court. I was terrified of court after my previous experience. We met the barrister from the insurance company at the accident scene early in the morning. Ted showed him the street, as I lay shaking in the car. We then drove to the court house. I was so ill I couldn't get out of the car, so Ted went to find out when I was needed. He said he would come and get me then. I suppose he would have had to carry me into the court room. After waiting for what seemed an eternity he returned to the car, leapt into the driver's seat and started the engine. He took me home to bed. Mr X had admitted liability on the court-house steps.

Relief at Mr X's admission of liability was both profound and gratifying. It was one thing that went right, one thing that made sense.

Once the first criminal case established that I was not responsible for the accident, I could start the long process of being assessed by doctors for the civil action. However the next few months proved that I was still like a puppet, powerless in a crazy world where I was forced by others to obey commands. This sensation of powerlessness continued through the round of doctors' visits necessary to prove that I was more than 30 per cent incapacitated. These were on top of all the doctors I had to visit to be assessed for Workcare and Transport Accident Commission requirements.

Even getting to the court steps was a mammoth task. I found

the build-up to the civil court case the very traumatic. I had eight different doctors to visit in just a few weeks. I saw three psychiatrists in one week, all of whom gave me the same IQ test. As a teacher, I knew that this test was invalid if taken more frequently than once a year! There was one psychiatrist who became very hostile and yelled at me, accusing me of cheating because I could do parts of the test easily and had difficulty with the mathematical parts.

A letter advising me to attend a series of doctors' appointments at various widespread locations arrived. The cost of taxis to these medical appointments and consultations was to be covered by the Transport Accident Commission. The visits were like some sort of macabre lucky dip. As each doctor was to write a report on my condition the consultations were frequently long and laborious. It was traumatic finding my way around by taxi, locating the doctor's rooms in the maze of hospital corridors and arriving on time in my bewildered, dazed state. On more than one occasion I was treated unkindly.

The inference appeared to be that I was a nuisance, a cheat and a liar. Rarely did I feel like a human being after sessions where I was ordered or even yelled at, to bend or move. Sometimes tests would be repeated many times until the doctor had gained proof that I was capable of producing a result through forced short-term repetition. It appeared to be of no interest or consequence to them that for the next few days I would be in severe pain.

At times, especially with tests where you had to put blocks or patterns together, the doctor would place the puzzle together, then push a block a quarter of an inch apart and ask me to complete the test. If I had coached my students as I was coached, they would have all come out as geniuses on tests!

I often didn't understand what was going on. One day I had to visit both a psychologist and a bone specialist. For some reason I had it firmly fixed in my mind that the first doctor was the psychologist, when he was in fact the bone man. It sounds crazy, but it was an example of how I didn't need to get much wrong to get it *all* wrong. For over an hour I answered all his questions as if he was a psychiatrist. It didn't occur to me that he wasn't. With enormous difficulty I convinced myself that his questions were based on psychiatry. I was perplexed when he spent so long examining my chest X-rays. Was this some kind of trick he was playing? I even commented to him that he appeared to understand a lot about bones! I took off my clothes as instructed and let him prod and feel my back and front. All this time warning bells were sounding in my head that things weren't 'quite right' because a psychologist shouldn't get you to take off your clothes.

It was not until I reached the next doctor who introduced himself, and explained that he was a psychologist, that the penny dropped. So I'd just seen the bone specialist. This explained the ghastly trouble I had trying to answer his questions. I had been so confused and so full of frustration. I would not have dared to ask for an explanation as to why he was examining me as he was. This episode left me feeling miserable and foolish.

I was amazed at the number of times long and laborious eye tests had to be completed. It was most distressing as the sight from my left eye was starting to be blocked out by my adjusting brain.

On another day, it was fortunate that Ted drove me to the consultation and waited in the car. Meanwhile the psychiatrist, in a very short time, had decided I needed to be committed to a mental institution, immediately hospitalised and drugs administered for my depression. What I needed was explanation and empathy, not being locked away! In my fragile state it was extremely difficult to walk out on an expert, a professional who had so quickly decided on such a drastic action. He even suggested I go straight from his rooms to the clinic, and that the family should bring in the things I needed after I had signed myself in. I felt shocked and powerless, and I was very lucky that Ted was waiting for me in the car that day.

The whole experience of repeatedly travelling and waiting

and trying to explain to my difficulties to yet another stranger was very damaging to both body and spirit.

By the time my civil action was to go to court my medical bills had reached over $50,000. Apart from the physio, osteopath and my local GP, the initial hospital stay, neurologist, strabismus surgeons, neuropsychologist, cardiologist, orthopaedic surgeon and ophthalmologist my GP had referred me to, the bulk of the money had been spent getting me assessed. None of the assessments had made me any better, if anything, the strain of the appointments had made me feel worse.

I'd never had anything to do with courts before, and had not realised that there are two different courts and their outcomes are based on different notions. The criminal court where the police had taken Mr X, had to prove things beyond a reasonable doubt, whereas in the civil court balance of probability is the main focus. If you are the person responsible for the accident, you cannot sue anyone. If only this were more generally known I'm sure people would take greater care and be more responsible on our roads.

Helen tried to explain the court system to me, but at the time I was not capable of understanding or remembering the points. Only now can I understand and see the relevance of what she was saying. If only I could have understood these things at the time I would not have felt so out of my depth in a crazy, mixed up world. Preparations for my civil case commenced a year after the accident. The case was eventually heard four years after the accident (apparently this is very fast for such an action). Helen wrote down the steps of a civil case for me. They were:
1. Make an appointment to see a solicitor — make sure it is a large firm that specialises in your area.
2. For the interview, bring along copies of all relevant documentation, and listen to the questions carefully. Answer any questions your solicitor may have and follow things up by letter. Remember to keep copies of everything

you pass on to the solicitor, and try not to give her too many documents.
3. Procedures go before the court. Barristers are now involved.
4. Court. Firstly you are listed for court. The list may be called over. There may be too many cases timetabled for court, so your case is put off to another day.
5. Then it is time for your day in court. Australia has an adversarial system, which means having to fight one side to disprove what the other side says.

I was beside myself with exhaustion because as well as my two half days a week at school, I had to travel to and locate out-of-the-way doctors' rooms for these medical appointments. On more than one occasion I found myself sobbing in the gutter when trying to get a taxi home.

Like a wounded animal, all I wanted to do was to be left alone at home with my pain and confusion. But I knew if I didn't co-operate by attending these medical appointments, things would be very grim for my court case. I felt traumatised because I was compelled to complete tests that reiterated my difficulties and not my strengths. I felt like screaming 'I don't want to be here! I just want to go home! Leave me alone!'

However, two doctors were kind and helpful. They explained some of my difficulties, which helped to fill in the jigsaw puzzle a little more.

One specialist, David de Horne, suggested that I visit the scene of the accident and place some flowers there. No-one had suggested such a thing to me before, but the idea really appealed. So, on the fourth anniversary of the accident Ted and I returned to the scene. He stayed in the car while I ventured out in the rain with some gold ribbon and roses. I put my arms around that pole, near the blue paint from my car that was still there. I tied the ribbon around the pole, then tucked the bunch of roses into the ribbon and spoke to the pole and thanked it for not taking my life. I planted a soft kiss where my hard car had been smashed. When I got back into the car to join Ted, my cheeks were wet, not only from the rain. From that moment I felt something inside me start to heal.

The civil case was listed to take place on a Monday nearly four years after the accident. On the Friday before the case, Ted was interstate on business and I was home alone when there was a phone call. An offer, an out-of-court settlement, was made. Apparently if I refused this offer and lost the court case, I might be offered less money and I would have to pay the costs of going to court. I panicked. What should I do? At last I managed to locate Ted at an airport on his way home. Even though my diligent and helpful barrister was confident we would get a better payout if we went to court, I felt that a bird in the hand was worth two in the bush. I was also afraid I might just die of fright in court. So I rang and accepted the settlement.

Now this civil case which had consumed so much of my time and energy was over, my first thought was to thank my lawyers. I managed to walk down the hill to the florist shop. Now it was my turn to buy flowers from this florist who had delivered so many beautiful bouquets to me. I took a taxi into the city to deliver the two huge arrangements, then Ted and the family met me and we celebrated with a late afternoon tea.

However when I got home exhaustion set in and my elation evaporated. I didn't feel so good about it all now. At dusk I slipped down into the garden and hugged the cool grey bark of a large lemon-scented gum, so like the telegraph pole, sobbing and begging, 'I'll give you back the money if you give me back my life!'

In the following weeks there was pleasure in giving some money to the kids so they could get something special, a reward for all they had done for me. I could spoil Ted, too and for myself I bought a warm winter's coat for standing in the street and waiting for taxis and a beautiful ring. There was a lot of thought behind the purchase of this ring. It was something I would have with me all the time. I had told myself then that the next time I felt like crying with frustration or self-pity I was to admire the ring instead. It was a celebration that I had a new start in life, a symbol that good can come from bad.

With the end of the court cases I thought that I would be free from appointments, that I would no longer have to see doctors if I didn't want to. But I found that financial advisers had taken their place. I had to be careful and wise in investing the money as my future looked different now I could only work part-time. The settlement money had to subsidise my salary. Helen told me that a large proportion of people who receive lump-sum payments go through their money within a few years.

 In retrospect, being upset by the reactions of other people was a dark place in the labyrinth

I was puzzled and perturbed by the reaction of some people to the fact I'd had a bad car accident. So many people were kind and considerate. However people demanded to know *why* I had the accident, perhaps to blame me or to make sure they don't make the same mistake.

Yet other people seemed relieved to learn that I was not to blame, that it was someone else's fault, that it was bad luck. Trying to understand this reaction made me think that they believed there was only so much bad luck floating around, and so if I had had bad luck, then there was less bad luck around to happen to them!

I was shocked that some people reacted in a way that showed they thought people got what they deserve. Therefore I must have deserved this accident!

Another reaction that upset me terribly was when people said things like: 'It is all for the best'; 'It was meant to be'; and 'It will all work out well in the end.'

Some of these reactions made me wonder if people are more primitive and superstitious than we think. Were these ways of showing sympathy or merely desensitising, coping strategies? Unfortunately these reactions made me feel confused and guilty.

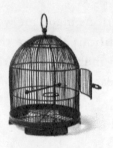

17.
As time goes by

'And in today already walks tomorrow.'
— Samuel Taylor Coleridge

Two summers came and went. We'd float on the swimming pool at the bottom of the garden, quietly watching ducks and water birds call in to drink. On hot evenings we'd dine with the kids on the deck with candles flickering in the trees. As time passed it was possible to become more reflective about the accident and change.

Apart from visits to doctors, school, physio and my parents, all my time was spent at home. Ted or the children would assist me to shop for food. After two years I could walk for ten minutes down the hill to the shop for milk, but had difficulty carrying it home and my shoulder and ribs would hurt the following day.

My friends were wonderful and visited me often to have coffee in the glass-room. After two years my dear friend Joyce decided that going out for coffee would do me good. So she drove me to a coffee shop. It was great to get out. After we'd enjoyed our coffee and a chat I decided that instead of troubling Joyce to drive me home I would walk the five kilometres home. I hated to be a nuisance and was petrified that a friend would be involved in an accident as a result of helping me. I didn't want to burden the family with whinging, and I felt self-indulgent with my complaints. Writing helped me cope with frustrations and sadness. That day I recorded:

> 'The walk home from Eltham was interesting. Bare hawthorn hedges cascaded with birds silhouetted against the evening sky, yesterday a glory of colour, now stark branches. The silence and solitude of the track, the little wooden bridge over the brown rushing waters of the creek trembles as I pass. I tap my way by peaceful fields of artichokes fringed with gum trees along the creek. I'm climbing up the hill now, with glimpses of the blue-mauve of the distant mountains against the pale lemon sky. Then I stumble down a steep slippery slope along the fence beside the horse paddock. Lights are starting to twinkle in the valley. How often must my feet tread this path? How often must my stick tap-tap this track? How frequently must my gloved hand fumble to touch a tree, a post, a branch searching for reality in this double world of mine? Oh Mr X, at the start of my walk home I cursed you, tears splashed down my face as car after car sped by me on the main road. I felt like an outcast — everyone else could drive. But to walk through the beauty of the valley has made me aware how wonderful (and fragile) life is.'

Another day I wrote:
> 'When trying on shoes today I had to ask the shop assistant to put the shoe on my left foot. No matter how hard I tried I just couldn't control my left leg. It felt as if someone had given me their left leg, so of course I couldn't control it. This must be the same silly leg I don't know I've got when I have a shower, so I don't remember to dry it afterwards. Then I try to push the wet thing out of bed. I wish I could get my own left leg back again!'

Some acquaintances would say with just a touch of jealousy 'What do you do with all the time on your hands?' 'I'm busy with doctors and physios and resting to get better', I reply. I often thought of my unhappiness and frustration, and my passion to return to an active life like theirs. Change places with me, please! I couldn't talk about the silly little happenings that would drive me crazy as I was so dependent and constrained. So I wrote:

> 'Today I stood in a hardware shop as tears ran down my cheeks like the rain running down the window from the cloudburst outside. Some dam burst in my head. Why was I crying? It was not that I had waited patiently 30 minutes for a taxi or waited patiently for another taxi just an hour before. Or that I'd waited patiently for the physio to use his magic hands to take away the pain for a few hours. It was the frustration of being powerless, of being trapped, of having no way out of this predicament. I could not change things by working or reasoning or creative thinking. All I could do was to find more patience. When the taxi eventually arrived the driver had just finished a cigarette, so I sat in the smelly stuffy taxi for a frenetic, fast and furious trip home.'

I had tried to set myself attainable goals. That day I would walk from the physio's to the shops five minutes away. I would carefully cross the road to the hardware store to buy some glue for my cracked walking stick. I would cross the road again and buy a fresh iced bun for Ken and Rob to have for morning tea. Not much of a goal, but as I stood in the hardware shop with the storm outside, I knew I couldn't face crossing the road again, so I wouldn't get a bun to proudly present to my boys, to put a smile on their faces. Instead they had to mop up my face.

I think one of the most frustrating and upsetting things about the whole situation was the never-ending snowballing effect of having a damaged body. You never knew where the next ache or pain would come from. If you drag your leg, you get muscle spasm pains in the foot. Because you can't judge heat or distance, you constantly burn or hurt yourself — I was always nursing a cut or burn or bruise. After two years I bent down one day and my lower rib twisted out, just like a powerful snake. It felt like it would poke right through my skin. A visit to my GP and physio followed. I saw a bone surgeon who suggested that he remove the offending rib. I didn't want that. I've since discovered that if I extend one leg out in the air when bending down — rather like a ballet dancer — the build-up of force on my diaphragm is released, and the rib stays where it is. Of course I sometimes forget and the rib pops out, catching me unawares.

I was in danger of becoming bitter and at times I still wondered whether life was worth living after having so much freedom and choice taken away. A great strain had been placed on Ted and the family. Then Rob, our youngest, was diagnosed with type I diabetes. Were the stresses and concerns caused by my accident to blame for this?

The accident occurred at the time when my career had the most potential. As the weeks passed I became more and more aware of my difficulties, and the hope that I would return to my classroom slipped just a fraction more from my grasp. I wrote in my journal:

'Am I a wimp? I have to steel myself to get into a car. I always ask myself 'Is this trip really worthwhile? Is it worth dying for?' Because I still have trouble understanding what people are saying, being with people makes me uncomfortable; music hurts my ears; familiar music reminds me I'm not the person I used to be; I can't read properly; I can't cope at the theatre or a movie; gardening's no good anymore; even walking is difficult with my balance and perception problems; watercolour painting is difficult; shopping and browsing are no longer a pleasure as I knock into people and things; the noise in restaurants means we have to eat out early to avoid the crowds and I still spill food, or miss my mouth, or dribble down my chin. Life is grim.

Giving up my committee work with Life Education and Philosophy for Children made me very sad. It's good to continuing teaching philosophy and extension work three mornings a week, but what is to become of me in the future? There is so much uncertainty in my life I feel I'm losing my nerve. I must be a wimp!

At first I thought getting better would happen naturally, like day follows night. It has been the bitterest pill to swallow to realise I will never be who I was. I don't know how much more improvement I can hope for. The accident has totally changed my capability to do the things that used to give me pleasure. It has also changed the amount of pleasure I get from doing those things I am still able to! Am I a very unlucky lucky person or a very lucky unlucky person?'

 In retrospect, being home alone and not knowing what to do was a dark place in the labyrinth

I was totally unprepared for the boredom and loneliness of being home alone. I'd spent my entire life being busy, interacting with other people at school, studying, working, raising a family etc. There had always been a focus to my life. Suddenly I was cut off from life, work and society. I'd always been a workaholic and now I didn't know how to distract myself. I didn't know how to live without my usual tasks and distractions.

I needed to have order in my day, to prioritise and break tasks into separate chunks, to write things down, to take notes during conversations so that I could follow the thread of the discussion, and to prepare notes in point form helps me cope with discussions with family and at work.

ORGANISING MY TIME

I tried to remember that exhaustion was never very far away. I tried to have a structured routine. A calm, well-organised environment really helped. I learnt to accept the fact that I only had an hour or two a day when I felt good, when I could achieve things. I've found that two decades after my brain injury I still need a nap.

DOING SOMETHING I LIKE EACH DAY

Each morning I needed to plan to do something that gave me pleasure each day. Unfortunately I didn't know what gave me pleasure. I should have kept a list on the fridge to refer to when I couldn't think of something pleasurable to do.

DOING SOMETHING TO HELP SOMEONE ELSE

I needed to figure out something to do to be helpful. Setting the table, unpacking the dishwasher and walking to the letterbox to get the mail gave me a sense of achievement but there must have been other things I could have done.

KNOWLEDGE

I had to remember that things weren't always simple. Coping with all the issues of brain injury is complicated. I needed to find out about brain damage and the different ways people cope with their challenges. I needed to learn about emotional healing, and how to cope with my grief and loss.

SIMPLICITY

I needed someone to help me to simplify issues and tasks by breaking them into small manageable chunks (although I might not have actually listened to them!).

PEACE AND QUIET

I found I had to have a silent house (no radio etc) to eliminate distractions. Noise made it impossible to absorb information. I did discover that at parties and family gatherings I preferred to sit on my own in a separate room and maybe talk to someone there.

NOT GIVING IN

I tried to remember to tell myself: 'When the going gets tough the tough get going'; 'If at first you don't succeed try and try again'; and 'There is no failure except in no longer trying'.

 In retrospect, not knowing what to do when I was overwhelmed by emotions and worries was a dark place in the labyrinth

Here is an alphabet of things I needed to do to help to relieve the pressure.

>   Appreciate something
>   Bawl: have a good cry
>   Call up a friend
>   Drink a coffee
>   Escape from it with a movie, TV or story
>   Focus on doing something
>   Get information
>   Hang onto hope. Home was my sanctuary.

Invest in the future — try to study something new
Jealousy was ruining my life
Knit, sew, do things with my hands
Laugh
Make things happen
Nothing stays the way it is - remember this
Observe how others have coped
Pray and Plan for something
Question
Run, walk, be physical
Spoil myself – do something nice
Talk about it
Understand my condition
Very positive attitudes help
Walk it away
eXorcise the demons lurking inside by bringing them out into the light
Yell, curse and let off steam
Zzz (sleep)

 In retrospect, being pessimistic was a dark place in the labyrinth

I realise now that hope, resilience, optimism and coping all come from one thing — how we think!

For my presentations I have done quite a bit of reading about pessimism and optimism and learnt that optimistic people bounce back more quickly from negative events. My lack of optimism certainly held me back.

Pessimistic people they don't take risks, or responsibility; they blame others; they are suspicious and oversensitive; they have difficulty concentrating; and they need constant reassurance and rewards. I realise now that I ticked all these boxes for the first few years after my accident. I was a walking, talking example of pessimism!

I was interested to learn that pessimistic people react to

setbacks by thinking they will last forever, that defeat in one area means defeat in all areas and that any setback is all their fault. That was me to a T! On the other hand optimists believe any setback is temporary, controllable and the result of bad luck —it is not their fault.

This book is an example of an optimistic person (before the accident) becoming a very pessimistic person (no wonder the 'new' me didn't feel like the 'old' me!) and then reverting to how I used to be — optimistic.

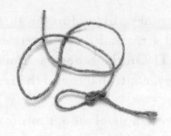

18.
Life goes on!

I've discovered that having a bad memory can be good — you can re-enjoy the same thing!
I've discovered that you can resent people who have power over you.

I suppose you could say I was thrashing round like a bee in a bottle, trying so hard to get better, to regain my lost life. I had an overwhelming determination to try to recapture as much of it as was humanly possible. I began to realise it would take longer than I hoped. In the past things had seemed straightforward, my goals attainable, shining on the horizon like the Emerald City in the Wizard of Oz. My road now had a big bend in it. The Emerald City could no longer be seen on the horizon; there were trees blocking any view of the horizon and my goals. Dangerous cliffs and rock slides on the road made every step forward a potential hazard. There were minefields all about me. At the same time I was scanning everywhere for an opportunity, or something that might lead the way to progress.

I still had the wonderful hours I spent at school. The remainder of my time was spent resting. I scribbled poems on scraps of paper to try to capture what was happening to my life. Trying to capture my experiences and express my thoughts was a challenge and gave me a sense of achievement. At least I was doing something, I was retraining myself to think and write. These brief poems and jottings assisted me in preparing for the doctors and lawyers and years later helped me put together the first draft of this book.

As each anniversary of the accident passed I found myself feeling sad that I wasn't 'better'. There was improvement, but in most cases, it was because I'd found ways of coping rather than the actual problem (sight, memory or pain for example) getting better. My energy was still being drained by my condition and the constant pain.

I was obsessed in trying to improve, and Dad encouraged me to try to identify the numerous problems that really upset me, and then try to understand how I could do something about it.

I realised that even if I didn't get better it was up to me to find ways to nibble away at the edges of problems until they were bearable. Just trying to improve helped me. But I must confess that in the deep recesses of my mind I was still wishing for a miracle — that I'd wake up one morning and I would be able to see properly, that a new doctor would have a new solution, or that my pain would melt away.

The black eye patch was driving me crazy. When I was out and about people would stare at me so I asked my optician if there was such thing as a contact lens with an eyeball painted on it that would block out the vision in the left eye. He did some investigating and found out about a business, several hours by plane away, that did such a thing. Ted and I travelled to the workshop to consult with them. A couple of weeks later my 'third eye' arrived. After I had gotten used to the contact lens I was feeling much less obvious out in public, but I was having a lot of accidents because I got no warning of impending danger coming from my left side and a strange milkiness would cloud my vision when I removed the painted contact lens.

Further investigation revealed that because of the paint on the lens my eye could not breathe and was being starved of oxygen; if

I continued using the lens I'd go blind in that eye. Then Helen rang me from work, she was very excited because she discovered that one of her clients also had a blocking-out third eye. A few days later she rang me from work. This time she was upset. The police had contacted her as her card was in the pocket of the man. He'd been run down and killed by a tram. The tram was coming from his 'blocked-out' side. That did it. My 'third eye' went in the bin.

I then decided to try dark tinted sunglasses for when I was out and about. I painted black inside the left lens. This allowed me to still have peripheral vision out the side of the glasses, to help avoid walking into vehicles, walls and people.

A disturbing facet of my faulty vision was that I could not recognize an object if I was looking down at it. Also, I could not gauge steps and distances. An object, say a tin of cat food, would be before me in the fridge but I would not be able to recognize it unless I bent down and had the object level with my face. To get a saucepan out of the cupboard required kneeling or lying on the floor so that my eye was level with the shelf. I could then see and recognise objects, but my knees then became a problem. Every gain seemed to have a corresponding loss, but I was learning to find ways to cope.

Yet I was as out of control of my situation as someone is on a rollercoaster ride. My behaviour flipped to extremes. Most of the time I was remote and meek, but sometimes I would shock myself by suddenly swearing, ranting and raving and crying. At other times I would just try to ignore the problems and pretend life was normal. Not wanting to be a nuisance to family and friends, I found myself withdrawing from the world. At other times I would try to concentrate on the positive or look for relaxing diversions, but finding relief in this way proved elusive.

Ted and I did manage to briefly escape everyday life with some breaks away. As I hated being in a car, flights to Sydney or Canberra were better diversions. However even though I felt safer in a plane than a car, there were a couple of issues. I would experience strong panic about being stuck in the plane while people queued up to exit. And whenever the plane would tilt taking off or landing, I would feel doubly disorientated as the effect added to my already unsteady sense of balance. I found that looking at something close to my face helped to block out the tilting world. Overnight stays in the country or seaside were a lovely break from routine. It was a real bonus to be away from home and not having to walk to the shops, or call for cabs, or have to deal with doctors or physios.

The family had their own ways of coping. Rob said the effect of the accident on him was like a whip that made him recoil. He socially withdrew, stunned and confused. He didn't ask the common question 'Why has this happened?' Instead he seemed to accept it on one level and gradually sort out the issues over a long period of time. Ann was busy running the house, she was doing so much to help, being both cook and bottle-washer, nurse and cheer squad. Ken and Helen had their uni life and studies to escape to, and Ted's time was taken up with a very hectic workload at work, and a stoic belief that we just had to hang in there.

After two years we realised that recovery was going to take longer than we'd all thought. Predictably it also had its ups and downs. I fell down, I got up, put a Band-Aid on my bleeding knees and struggled on till my next fall.

My 50th birthday turned out to be during a time I was better than I had been, but still feeling very miserable. Birthday celebrations at home are always doubled in pleasure in our household, as Ted's birthday falls on the day after mine. The Friday of my birthday dawned wet, chilly and dreary — fairly much in tune with how I felt — depressed and aching. I'd been wrestling with one of my nasty and numerous chest infections for a couple of weeks.

As a treat, the whole family was to spend the night at Queenscliff. After an Aspro Clear cocktail that afternoon, Ken drove me to the city where Ted picked me up for our big adventure. Off we went, full of optimism. We arrived at our destination in a flurry of squalls and dashed from the dreadful weather to the warm, welcoming, lit and orderly Queenscliff Hotel. It was bliss.

Orchids from an old school friend were in our room. There was a joyous festive feeling as the family gradually took over the first floor, safely in from the cold. Ted produced an exquisite ring; what a surprise and a thrill! The whole family gathered in front of a roaring fire in the front parlour. I felt like a queen going into the beautiful candle-lit dining-room surrounded by the jewels of our family. After dinner we sat in the charming sitting-room where the kids played chess and card games. Outside the storm raged. Inside we were cosy and cheery. We had weathered the storm.

In another highlight Helen and Greg's wedding was celebrated at Montsalvat the following year. The early morning sun glowed through the beautiful old windows as they stood barefoot and crowned with garlands — a joyous happening. Ann and Tony were wed a year later at dusk, also at Montsalvat. The dark pool was twinkling with dozens of floating candles and strains of jazz played through the starlit velvet sky.

Mum and Dad were there for the weddings. The family was together. Wonderful.

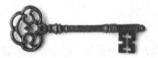

19.
Examining the heart

'Take away love and our earth is a tomb.' Robert Browning
(Wo)'man — a being in search of meaning.' Plato
'Ignorance is never better than knowledge.' Enrico Fermi

Seeing and facing the facts came in many forms. One sunny afternoon Ted and I were out and about and we began browsing in a bookshop. Ted was engrossed so I decided to try to select a book to read. I'd read only a couple of books in the past few years, but perhaps I could rediscover the bookworm side of me. What book could I choose? Not one about travel; if you can't travel, you're no longer interested in the subject, and travel was a reminder of the 'old' me. I searched through the other books but there were no paperbacks with print large enough for me to read and I didn't want crime, anything frightening or sad either.

Suddenly it hit me. Just like Jenny, the mother of one of my pupils who was very ill with cancer, I'd lost my interest in reading. If the subject matter was too shallow, it didn't feel worth the struggle, on the other hand, serious subject matter seemed too real, too upsetting and disturbing. This revelation brought to the surface the sadness and frustration that was bubbling, almost out of control, beneath the surface of my life and made me face reality — I hadn't really come to terms and I wasn't really coping emotionally with my changed life. I had spent years pretending that I was okay, but I now realised I had to take off my mask and confide in Hugh, my wonderful GP. After some discussion he referred me to a psychologist. He said she was a delightful lady and that we should get on well together.

My first visit to June the psychologist left me seething! I tried frantically to sweep my sadness under the mat and deny that I was lost and depressed. 'I'll never come back, so there!' I kept telling myself as I sat through our first session. My homework was to write down things that gave me some pleasure. 'What a stupid thing to do — nothing gives me pleasure!' I thought.

Later, as I was sitting on the deck having a cup of coffee I realised that even though I couldn't smell or taste the coffee, holding the warm mug in my hands felt good! The sun on my back felt good! Goodness me! I grabbed a pencil and paper and started to jot down things that gave me pleasure. My list included: Ted and the kids being home, achieving anything, nature, having a hot shower for the pain, tapestry, drinking coffee in the sun, feeding the birds and having Steff, our dog, by my side. Wow! This was amazing! Even if some things were fairly insignificant, there was some pleasure in my life of pain.

I took that list and another list of things that perplexed me, to my next appointment: I could not remember my way around my own house; I couldn't find the tap to turn off the hose; I keep expecting Rob to be ten, not seventeen; I felt trapped, disempowered and dependent; my career was gone; I was pushy with the family; I felt I didn't belong at school; I was angry and frustrated and felt as if I was just going through the motions with life; everyone, including me, expected me to be better by this time, but I wasn't; and I felt I was constantly disappointing everyone.

I learnt that I had three main issues to resolve: firstly, I had to stop pretending that I was happy when I wasn't, and that I understood people when I didn't. Secondly, I needed to stop being constantly disappointed in myself. Thirdly, I needed to find ways to deal with my constant frustration.

June pointed out that my struggle to recapture my old self was taking too much of a toll. My grief was being protracted by trying to retrieve my old self because so much of my emotional energy was going into the battle to become more like I was in the past. I needed to try to redefine myself but this notion terrified me. My mental changes in memory, retrieving words, the concept of number etc (rather than cognitive functioning, which seemed intact) had had a devastating effect on my day-to-day life, and I needed to find new things to enjoy that I could achieve. I had to try to accept myself as I was, to look for a new career, and to be content with nibbling around the edges of my trauma. Knocking off little bits at a time helped to lighten the weight, and I slowly learnt to cope by breaking up big tasks into small, more manageable ones.

As for my panic attacks, I couldn't do anything in the middle of an attack. I just had to wait for the adrenalin rush to pass. Over time I learnt to go into a shop and ask for bread or bananas without crying, and to find my way to and from doctors' appointments in the city without panicking.

But it was one sunny morning when June made the most helpful suggestion. She said 'Chris, what would you say if I said a friend from work had head injuries and was experiencing all the problems you have outlined to me?' I thought for a second then said 'Of course I would say how sorry I was that they had difficult challenges. I'd tell them it's okay, to slow down, that their mistakes don't matter'. June then said something quite startling. She said I had to learn to treat the damaged side of myself — the one I called my bumbling idiot — as if she was my own best friend! Instead of being hostile and critical of this other me, I was to try to be kind and helpful. I was to say in my head things to my best friend. If I forgot something I'd say 'Don't worry, next time let's write that down, let's make a list'. When I broke something, I'd say 'everyone breaks things, it's not that big a deal'. These conversations helped to calm me down, and also broke me of the habit of seeing things as symbols that I was no longer any good.

It was wonderful to have June to talk about how I was mad and stupid. One day I looked out the window and although it wasn't raining I could see water falling on one part of the garden. Wow! I thought, this is weird and exciting! I returned to the window to look at the garden several times over the next half-hour or so. What was happening? Should I ring the newspaper to get someone to witness this incredible phenomenon? I then forgot the whole episode and later when I went to the letterbox, I saw that the hose was on. It took me a few minutes to realise that *this* had been the magic rain from heaven!

Another day I saw circles on the gravel drive. A similar flood of wonderment and trying to make sense of the occurrence happened in my head. Could it be visitors from outer space? Were the circles made by the same creatures that made the circles in the crops in England? Yet again the hose was the culprit.

At school one day I noticed a mother talking to a tree. 'Oh the poor thing! I wonder if she is okay? What should I do? Take her to the principal? Go and make her a cup of coffee? How can I help?' After what seemed a long time exploring possibilities, her friend, who was standing *behind* the tree, moved into view. Little episodes like these confirmed to me I was mad and stupid. I knew that normal people don't jump to conclusions like this!

June said my problem was the creative side of my brain taking over. She said that if anything seemed weird or odd I had to check all the information available and go back to something I understood. I had to look at the *facts* and widen my knowledge base before coming to a conclusion. In retrospect, I believe these were all indications of my incredibly one-tracked mind. It was so hard to understand or form thoughts that any distraction would mean I entirely lost what I was saying or thinking. My way of coping was to hang onto an idea for grim life!

So gradually my 'best friend' and I learnt to increase our

enjoyment in things. Progress was measured according to what I had achieved in a week or a month. According to June I seemed to have only two speeds — motionless or flat out fast. Looking after my best friend let me try an alternative way of looking at things (when I remembered to do so).

Disorientation in the morning still troubled me greatly. I would wake up not knowing who I was or what day it was. Somehow this seemed like personal proof that the bumbling idiot had taken over my body. It took me many years to be able to wake up and say, 'Today is Thursday. On Thursdays I do this and this'. Ted found it strange when I lay in bed some mornings looking upset and puzzled just because I didn't know what day it was. He'd reassure me, 'You shouldn't worry — I'll *tell* you what day it is each day'. But that was not the point. I needed to *do things for myself*. As with so many problems, the solution ended up being a simple one. I put a page-by-page calendar by my bed that I could turn over each morning to see the day and schedule.

Taxis were another trauma on my list. I'd go out to a doctor's appointment and use the opportunity to shop, then push myself so hard while I was out and about that before I knew it I'd be over my threshold of tiredness. This explained why I had spent miserable times sitting in the gutter, sobbing as if my heart was broken, all because I couldn't get a taxi! June suggested that I always have a plan for getting a taxi. When I'm in the city I can go to a taxi rank at any of the large hotels. If no taxi comes to the rank, I go and sit down, have a rest, *then* try again. Even though sometimes it felt like the end of the world, and all I wanted was *bed*, it wasn't the end of the world and I could find a way to cope.

I also carried a list in my bag entitled 'What to do when I don't know what to do'. Suggestions included: sit down, don't panic, ring Ted or Ken, always keep a phone card or coins for the phone, especially for a taxi. This was such an obvious thing, but I actually needed June to point it out. I'd tried organising taxis ahead of time by pre-booking them but something would always disrupt the plan. Once I got a mobile phone, getting a taxi became much easier.

I believed June when she explained that school was taking up all my effort, but I still hung on the goal of staying in work for dear life!

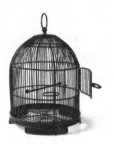

20.
Facing the music

I've discovered that believing is seeing (the way we see things, is affected by what we believe.)
I've discovered that seeing is believing (sometimes we can only believe something if we see it or read about it.)

We used to have a darling brown poodle called Beaver Brown. On the day we bought him we took him to the beach where he delighted the children with his antics: tumbling cutely into the depressions in the sand, chasing seagulls and displayed curiosity in everything. That night, as we were tucking Beaver Brown up with his hot water bottle and clock, we saw he was having trouble breathing.

'Oh no,' we thought, 'we've been sold a sick pup!'

So we made an after-hours visit to the vet. To our astonishment, the vet took a pair of tweezers and started to pull at a tiny splinter, no thicker than a hair, which he'd noticed in Beaver Brown's neck. He pulled and pulled, and to our shock, out came a three-inch long grass seed. It was just like watching a magician doing a trick. We gaped at this seed that had worked itself into Beaver's flesh. How thankful we were that we'd taken the dog to the vet that evening. By morning his throat may have become so swollen he could have choked. That grass seed was invisible, unimagined, yet so dangerous!

June found the tiny tip of an idea-seed poking out of me. It took many months talking with her before this secret seed that was growing so deep beneath the surface poked a tentative shoot into the light of day. It was an example of what you believe influences how you see.

Ted had been *wonderful*. Ted had done so much for me. Ted had changed his life to revolve around me and there was daily evidence of his care for me, but I was blind to all these facts. Because I felt so pathetic, hopeless and helpless, guilty, ashamed and disgusted in myself I believed that *no-one* could possibly love me. I was not the girl he'd married 27 years ago, nor was I the wife he had before the accident. So I became fixated on looking for proof that he didn't love me! I became totally absorbed by the idea that, 'If he loved me he would do what I wanted'.

When I thought of an example of how he didn't love me I secretly wrote it down. I ended up with a list: if he really loved me he would have sat beside me when I was in hospital; if he really loved me he wouldn't have let me be tortured by the physio or left me in the hospital in the multi-bed ward; if he really loved me he wouldn't have poked that overcooked rubbery eight-minute microwaved egg into me and thought he'd helped me.

June suggested that I should talk about some these ideas that were affecting me so badly. Little did June know it but these ideas were actually breaking my heart! As a result of June's suggestion I eventually drummed up the courage to tackle these ideas one at a time. Tentatively I mentioned Ted's brief visits to hospital to the kids. They said in astonishment, 'Mum, Dad was with you the whole time you were in intensive care, he hardly came home'. But at that time I had been unconscious! I didn't know that he'd been with me! Oh dear! Once I was out of danger and conscious Ted would briefly visit me when he could on his way to and from work. I would lie there, thinking, 'His job is more important and has higher priority than me!'

So I spoke to Ted and learnt that he was just trying to hold on to his job, and make up for some of the time he had spent with the unconscious me! He was having trouble coping. He was also so shocked by all that had happened that he just wanted to escape from the hospital once he knew I was going to survive! As for having me shifted to another hospital, the thought hadn't entered his head because he thought I was receiving the best care I could get. He was a man of action. When he fed me the egg he thought was doing something to help!

June pointed out that it was lack of understanding, *not* lack of love, on Ted's part. But deep in the recesses of my mind I knew I had the *absolute* proof that Ted didn't love me! He had never given me a pat! For over two years I had yearned for a pat — more than air! Rob would sit by my side and pat my knee, but Ted had never given me a pat! One day, when we were in the garden picking some honesty plant, the plant seemed to say to me 'for heaven's sake be honest with Ted!' So I used all my courage to say 'Darling you don't really love me because you've never given me a pat!'

He was shocked and replied 'But a pat wouldn't make you better. I could get you a pillow or more painkillers, that might help, but a pat?' So we got to the heart of my sadness, and found we could discuss how differently we thought. I came to realise that Ted was not a mind reader.

I needed empathy, Ted needed to fix things.

Once this idea-seed was extracted, and I could examine it in the light of day, the painful swelling subsided and I could breathe, think and live anew.

What I believed had strongly influenced how I perceived things. Confusingly, at other times, the reverse was true: I could only believe in something once I had seen it, or someone else had seen it!

If pulling out the grass seed of an idea was a heart mender, my appointment with Dr Maureen Malloy was a key to open my mind. I had been sent to so many specialists. I never knew if they would have any solutions to my pain, sight or understanding problems. But this time I hit the jackpot — a wise, empathetic and understanding doctor. She treated me like a person, not a patient and she understood my difficulties! I had spent so many specialist visits trying to explain all my problems. Until I saw Dr Malloy, no specialist had appeared to understand the torment I was in. No one had explained that the symptoms I was experiencing were typical of head injury.

Dr Malloy showed me that seeing proof or evidence affected what I believed! After giving me a test she would look at the results. She would then translate the results into something I could understand. For example, because she understood problems arising from memory deficits she suggested that perhaps I had difficulty following conversations in the school staff room. Good heavens, this was true! I knew I felt uncomfortable in a group, that I found it hard, but I had not analysed why! My faulty short term memory was why I couldn't follow conversations!

Like a magician pulling rabbits out of a hat she explained many of the unseen and unspoken things that were a part of this new life I was trying to cope with. Instead of me trying to express my difficulties with this new life, here was someone who fully acknowledged the ramifications of the difficulties associated with brain injury. Just one hour spent with someone who really understood profoundly affected my general wellbeing.

The relief was immense. For several years I'd felt guilty about not getting better. This was in spite of constant effort to make things 'right', by acting and pretending I was ok, which involved sweeping many uncomfortable things under the carpet.

The main thrust of the help I had been given from professionals and people I'd meet, was for me to focus on the positive things in life — I was lucky to be alive and lucky to be not more seriously injured. Looking back I can see I was obviously depressed, lost and bewildered, totally swamped by the negative. I couldn't even remember to focus on the positive! Even when I did, I found that just thinking positively didn't help me walk, tell the time, or cope. I needed to understand.

Dr Molloy explained that my thoughts had been flowing too quickly for my memory to keep up, and she gave me strategies for coping with this strange world I found myself in.

1. Touching things to help me focus.
2. If I was trying to remember something, to shut my eyes to visualise without distractions.
3. As I could only cope with small amounts of information, to break information into manageable chunks. This was so helpful: examples included focusing on one utensil at a time when setting the table, or breaking a telephone number into two or three digits at a time.
4. I needed time to get a meaningful idea in my mind.
5. I needed to set priorities:
- to learn be comfortable with myself
- to zipper my mouth so that I was not annoying and frustrating for my family through endlessly asking them to explain and repeat things
- to keep my thoughts to myself
- to remember that it doesn't matter if I miss out on some things — I do not need to be always struggling and fretting, trying to understand
- to be a willow and bend with life's forces, and not try to remain rigid and un-yielding.

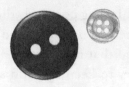

21.
Mum and Dad

'Their love was boundless, their adventurous spirit unquenchable, their sense of fun legendary and their creativity and wisdom only exceeded by their universal generosity.'
— Plaque on my parents' memorial rose bush

My parents were a constant source of support and hardly a day passed without some contact with them. They would often make the hour-long journey from their bayside home to try to encourage me. I feel so sorry that for the last four years of their lives my condition was a constant concern to them. Our visits to my childhood home for coffee and a chat around the table in the sunroom and a wander around the garden comforted me like nothing else.

These times were always an occasion for them. The smell of brewing coffee would greet us at the front door, ahead of Dad, with his arms wide open for a bear hug. There would always be something special, like freshly baked cream kisses or a piece of mellow cheese. Everything would be in readiness and it felt so good to be the highlight of their day. Even though they were elderly it somehow seemed okay for them to fuss and look after and spoil me. We'd leave with flowers from the garden and something to take home as a treat for the family.

Ted's parents had been neighbours and close friends of my parents for over 50 years. Ted's dad had died some years ago. His mum's health was not good and she had to be moved into a nursing home. Her life had been devoted to music. She had been my music teacher and confidant during my mum and dad's regular overseas visits. I'd had lessons at their home across the road. I can remember my hands sticking to the piano keys during lessons when Ted, on returning from school, would pop his head round the door to ask what there was to eat. Not the boy next door but the boy across the road!

The fourth year after my accident, Ted's mum died, and my mother's health was deteriorating to such an extent that Dad could no longer care for her at home. The week she was installed in a nursing home nearby, Dad was diagnosed with leukaemia. I still struggle with feelings of guilt because I was unable to be of much support to them during their final months. I would take a taxi to their home to spend some time with Dad, then Ted would take us to visit Mum.

Dad mastered using a computer at the age of 80, and wrote a wonderful book about his life. I wish I'd been able to read it, but reading was so difficult at the time. In retrospect, I could have asked Ted to read it to me, then Dad and I could have discussed it during the pleasant afternoons we shared together. We had wonderful philosophical discussions about life. He enjoyed telling me stories of his childhood. Some of his stories helped me to see a different, more positive view of life.

By a strange quirk of fate, Dad's favourite spot when he was lad living in Kew was by the Yarra River, only a few metres from where my accident occurred. I had thought of the spot with horror and it felt like an area of darkness until Dad told me of the thrills he'd had as a boy there when he'd see rows of beautiful Canadian canoes and rowing skiffs full of inviting colourful cushions for hire. He said as you floated down the river on a Sunday afternoon, you knew you were getting close to the boathouse as the sound of the gramophone came into earshot. Dad's memories changed my ghastly memories of that area.

Dad frequently spoke about his 'guardian angel' and my ears pricked up. I had my own — a flesh and blood one — Peter! There were times in Dad's life when his angel must have worked overtime. When he was about four, on holiday with his family in the hills at Belgrave, he found his father's Harrington & Richards shotgun in the wardrobe. Dad could hardly lift the gun let alone hold it to his shoulder. He was playing with it, making all the appropriate noises. His grandmother was in the living room reading when he pointed it towards her and said 'Bang Bang'. She said, 'Dear, take it away, I hate guns'. So he took it into the passage just six feet away, pointed it towards the back door and pulled the trigger and said 'bang' again. There was a terrific explosion; the recoil sent him hurtling backwards. The back door had completely vanished!

I was curious why Dad had titled his book *Like Ants of a Summer's Day*. He explained that when he was five his grandfather once remarked to him, 'Markie we are all just like ants of a summer's day' (meaning man's existence is brief and insignificant in the boundless universe). Dad had no idea of what the words meant but the way his grandfather treated him like a grown-up person left a lasting memory.

Considering all the factors that helped me to recapture my life, I believe the way my Dad always regarded me as an intelligent, thoughtful human being was most important. From the time when I was only five, Dad would treat me as an adult and take me on 'thinking walks'. We would discuss all sorts of things like politics, current affairs and opera. I certainly could not understand what Dad was talking about, but because he took the time and effort, to treat me as a grown-up, he lit a little flame of hope and belief in myself, that never got snuffed out.

Dad was always keen to discuss my lessons and give suggestions, and before long, school-day and teacher stories would follow. His earliest school days were sweetened by the words of encouragement Miss Grey (his teacher) gave, when she'd praised his plasticine sparrow. He had the pleasure of helping her with a hearing aid when she was an old lady and discovered that she regarded encouragement as the greatest gift a teacher could give.

Dad spoke constantly about people's great need for appreciation, approbation and encouragement. Encouragement had been a strong thread, like gold, woven through my life. It has helped me to cope. Encouragement was at the heart of another of Dad's stories. On a cold grey day (when I was a year old) Dad was wandering round the grounds of the US educational institution made famous by Helen Keller, when he was invited to observe a young lady teaching a sweet little girl who was deaf and blind. When he was leaving, he tried to express his admiration for the teacher's patience and skill. To his surprise the teacher burst into tears. She said that she was discouraged at the slowness of results, and was on the point of giving up, but that Dad's words had renewed her spirit. He said that the weather was even more dismal when he left the building but he felt like he was walking on air. 'Chick, we can never know the importance of words of encouragement'.

Dad met and spoke to Helen Keller. He would recount her famous words about how sometimes when we look at a door of happiness 'another opens; but often we look so long at the closed door that we do not see the one which has been opened for us'.

Mum had been in a nursing home for only three months when she fell and broke her hip, she then developed pneumonia. Dad spent a lot of time visiting her, and was being his usual busy self, preparing the Christmas cake and pudding the month before Christmas when he became desperately ill with an infection. Mum died several days later, on an afternoon when I was with her. Dad, who was in hospital receiving transfusions, passed away three days later.

At the funeral Mum and Dad were united in one coffin. We had baskets of oranges for guests to take as a memento of how they met — Mum's bag of oranges broke on the street, and Dad had stopped to pick them up for her.

In the cemetery their rose bush is just across a path from Ted's parents' grave. They are still neighbours.

It is only now a decade later that I recognise that so much of the way I have tackled my challenges are a result of the life philosophy of my parents. I was brought up with a can-do, we-can-find-ways-to-solve-problems attitude. From the time I was a small child I was surrounded by Mum and Dad's stories that carried the message that it was most important to be fiercely independent, to stand on my own two feet, to tackle my challenges head on, to have a go and to never give up.

Their stories held many examples from riding their push-bikes on a 500 kilometre round trip down the Great Ocean Road in the early days of their marriage, to later travelling up the Amazon River, sailing across Lake Titicaca or visiting leper colonies in Fiji at a time when adventure travel was rare. Their life was packed with tackling new experiences.

We would chuckle as Dad retold the stories of when he living on an isolated property in the mountains and running low on supplies, but was expecting an important visitor. As he had no milk for tea he'd watered down calcimine to be 'milk', and, needing an egg to make a cake, squeezed an egg out of a chook who was late in producing the morning egg. Dad was constantly inventing things. He devised one of the earliest Australian hearing aids. Mum was game for anything: she smuggled some women's magazines into the Soviet Union so that she could give them to women to show what life was like in the West; she would also give a lift in the car to any tramp or swagman standing by the side of the road.

This can-do attitude, which initially left me so desolate and feeling like a failure — hopeless and helpless — has, in the long run, helped me to experiment to try to find different ways to tackle my challenges.

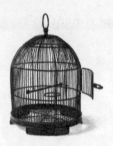

22.
The year of the dove

'There is nothing either good or bad but thinking makes it so.' Shakespeare
I've discovered that mind power is amazing.
I've discovered what doesn't kill you makes you stronger.

1996 Journal
'Today is the five year mark of that day when my life changed. I woke up feeling miserable and tried to work out why: for the past four years the accident anniversary has meant family celebrations that I survived. Suddenly I realised that I'd been telling myself "Be patient and you'll be better in the future!" My idea of the future was obviously five years! I certainly am not better!

At school I was feeling sorry for myself when Mimi sat down beside me and declared, "I love you!" The students were challenged and eager to share their discoveries about life for the 'Pearls of Wisdom' book we are making in our philosophy/thinking workshops. Their ideas captured my attention and imagination. Comments such as "I've discovered that the things you enjoy doing, you often do well"; "I've discovered that if you take your time you will make it"; "I've discovered that you don't feel as stupid if you make a mistake and others make the same mistake"; "I've discovered that you can't read people's thoughts"; and "I've discovered that I don't want to eat pickled eel's feet" made me smile and lifted my spirits — I learnt so much about life from my students.

On my way home in the taxi I reflected about how I've pushed myself but it has been worth it, I've accepted my changed life and learnt ways to cope. I still stumble, fall, and get lost, but apart from annoyance at the inconvenience, I don't berate myself for being dumb or stupid. I now get worn-out, so most days I take an afternoon nap. I know that if I don't nap I get over-exhausted and may need to take a sleeping pill at night, because I'm get over-exhausted, but that's okay, too. When I'm out, I find a seat and rest when I'm dog-tired. My mobile phone has made a huge difference because now I can ring for taxis easily. My shoulder and ribs are still very painful but a weekly visit to my osteopath helps my dizziness and keeps the pain at a level I can cope with. (I must admit though that I still have the sensation that I've got a tomahawk embedded in my back!) I now know to take care when bending or doing up shoelaces so that my lower ribs do not pop out. My double vision still drives me crazy but I haven't found the solution yet.

Love has pushed and pulled me to cope: the family's encouragement, patience, innovation and love have not only changed the world for me, but changed me for the world. I am so thankful for the understanding that developed after Ted and I eventually stopped sweeping things under the mat and discussed how we really felt. It is only now that I am starting to realise what he has gone through. I had been caught up in my own misery for so long, that I had not understood that he was angry, not at me, but angry because he was so frustrated to see me suffer. Understanding has strengthened our relationship, and he's been the wind beneath my wings. Long ago Ted once remarked "With all the best will in the world it requires a great degree of acrobatic expertise to make love to a woman with a smashed skeletal frame". We have proved with time, gentleness and love all things are possible. Ted says that the accident has helped him to prioritise issues, and showed him that relationships are the more precious thing in life.

Yesterday we'd stood on the deck watch a pair of superb king parrots breakfast from the bird feeding-tray. It was a foggy morning and the birds shone like two bright jewels floating in milk. Birds have been a happy thread running through my days. Five years ago, in my first agonising days at home, Ken had tried to interest me in a couple of tame white doves that had been pensioned off by a magician. This idea captivated my imagination — wouldn't it be wonderful to have a bird that was a symbol for peace, hope and magic to sit on my shoulder — not a parrot that I needed to complete the effect when I wore my eye patch! But all the magician's doves had been purchased. I was so disappointed that the kids decided that they would get me some doves.

For weeks they became architects and designed countless quaint, weird and amazing dovecotes. Time passed. The pile of design drawings grew, pages torn or photocopied from books and magazines joined the pile. This labour of love became a point of contention as no-one could decide the winning design for the Dove Taj Mahal. The whole idea was dropped. Secretly I felt let down. I didn't mind what the dovecote was like, I really fancied some doves!

Today Ken rang me so see if I was okay. He sounded very pleased with himself. Apparently there was a month-old fan-tail dove at the artist's colony of Montsalvat that was being pecked by the other birds in the aviary. Would I like it? Would I what! I jumped at the chance! Tonight Ken arrived home with a bedraggled, pathetic grubby white bundle of feathers in a cardboard box. It had no tail feathers yet, and because of the way it pushed up its chest when it tried to stand it had no balance. Oh, so like a white ghost of me five years ago.

It was love at first sight, and the little dove nestled up to me, sitting contentedly on my knee. When Helen saw us together she christened my new friend "Lovey-dovey".'

Lovey's tail became a beautiful snowy fan and Ken presented me with Cloud, another white fantail. At first Lovey spent much of the day with me, wrapped in a towel sitting on my knee. Later she'd sit on my shoulder and snuggle into my hair while I worked on this manuscript on the computer. I'd give her 'flying lessons' till she learnt to flap about then return to perch on my head or Steff's head — much to his surprise.

Fantails doves are handsome but clumsy. They flap and flutter awkwardly, and on the ground they waddle and shuffle in circles, frequently with their head down their back. As they can't see where they are going they fall down steps or off the deck railing. I'd say to them 'Oh you poor different things, you can't walk like an animal and yet you're not like a true flying bird'.

I was fascinated to find out why they were purposely bred like that; to fly up in the air and flap to cause a commotion for the homing pigeons to see so they can return safely home.

Like Lovey and Cloud, I too was awkward, ungainly and different. But my purpose in life and my writing is to point the way, to mark the spot so that people, not pigeons, can find understanding and peace after their long and arduous journey from the labyrinth of trauma and change that is brain injury.

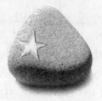

23.
Killing three birds with one stone

'What lies behind us and what lies before us are tiny matters compared with what lies within us'.
Framed notice in the office of Brooklyn Heights School

Weird and wonderful plants were starting to pop up in the garden where Lovey and Cloud had spilt their pigeon mix. At the same time a little shoot of an idea emerged from the dark recesses of my mind and grew until I became obsessed. If only I could find out more about brain injury and how people successfully cope, maybe *then* I'd understand and improve.

I seemed to have exhausted every possibility of discovery in Australia and I had unearthed some interesting information from the US. I'd reasoned that because there were more people in the US, there would be more people with brain injury and maybe more would be known about it. What's more, maybe there would be a doctor who could 'fix' my double vision! About this time Helen obtained a Queen's Scholarship and went to study for her doctorate in law at New York University. A visit to NY would kill three birds with one stone! It would be wonderful to see Helen as well as possibly providing me with answers to my questions. It didn't enter my head that to find the 'right' people to get the 'right' information was like a wild goose chase and could prove to be fruitless. I was just sure that a trip across the seas would prove helpful.

Helen greeted us at JFK airport and took us to her tiny apartment in Brooklyn Heights. It was wonderful to see her again and to explore the city with her. She'd chased down and made appointments with professionals associated with brain injury for us. One holiday weekend we took the train to Boston to see the autumn leaves. Every hotel had been booked out, but, after numerous phone calls we obtained lodgings at the John Jeffries House. Our taxi from the station took us through dark and rainy streets to the old rest-house.

We got to our room and I pushed back the curtains to look out into the night. The first thing that I saw was a large sign on the building across the street: Massachusetts Eye and Ear Infirmary. How incredible! Maybe someone there could help me. The literature in our room explained that the guest house was used by people visiting the Infirmary. 'Curiouser and curiouser' as Alice would say! After many phone calls and more than a little pushing I obtained an appointment for 9am the following morning with a Dr Azar, whose field of expertise was double vision.

Dr Azar understood the complexities of my vision. Apparently only a small number of doctors were likely to be *au fait* with my situation. Surgery might be a solution and there was one doctor in Australia who might be able to help me. His practice was just a half-hour drive from our home. I don't need to describe our delight or amazement.

Our trip to the US was proving to be successful and our luck continued when we returned from Boston to Helen's apartment. By making numerous calls to anyone we could trace who had anything to do with brain injury we learnt that the first meeting of the Brooklyn Chapter of the Head Injury Association would be held nearby that weekend. Ted and I attended the meeting and learnt that every 15 seconds someone in the US suffers a brain injury and that every year 500,000 to 700,000 people in the US require hospitalisation because of brain injury.

Dr John Ryder's speech proved we'd found a 'goose' in our wild goose chase. I whispered in Ted's ear, 'It was worth the trip just for these past 20 minutes!' as Dr Ryder used analogies to explain brain injury. For the first time I started to understand: he said that if New York was devastated by an earthquake it would be difficult to get across town with bridges down and fallen buildings blocking our way. We might eventually be able to reach our destination, but it would require a lot more time retracing our steps because of the lack of a bridge or avoiding fallen debris. He also likened brain injury to a vandalised telephone exchange where a whole city block is disconnected. This vandalism would have far-reaching ramifications. Communication would be scrambled and the brain taxed in trying to understand; what had been easy and automatic would become very difficult.

Dr Ryder spoke of the way brain injury disrupts how we process information — people with brain injury may feel ill at ease because even a simple task such as making and drinking a cup of tea may no longer be easy and routine. The person may make errors, be forgetful, drop or spill the tea, all of which could make them feel foolish and lose self-esteem.

He explained that:
- Brain injury is a lifelong problem. You need the support of family, friends and a good doctor.
- The brain will sprout new fibres with use. It will slowly regrow.
- You must work on things you have difficulty with.
- Things needn't look so dark because you can move on to a more fulfilling life.
- You must never give up.

His advice also included:
- Put in an effort because the more effort you put in the more you will recover.
- You need to adapt and learn new tricks.
- You need to slow down so that you become more aware and do things carefully.
- Relaxation is important.
- Noise can irritate and make you angry and stressed.
- You need to monitor yourself and become more aware of what's going on, and become aware of your strengths and personal resources.
- You need to build up your brain — to recognise the things that have gone (your weaknesses) and the things that you have (your strengths).

The next speaker, Deborah Fedor, had a brain injury which she likened to being plucked from Brooklyn and put in Greenland. She couldn't read, she got lost when she left the house and suffered great strain to her marriage due to communication problems. Deborah spoke about the general myths of brain injury — that people with brain injury can't think and that they're not intelligent.

Her advice was:
- To go outside rehab to improve. She'd gone to a nearby gym six days a week, plus she and her husband saw a marriage guidance counsellor who didn't know about brain injury but could help them with their miscommunication problems.
- Brain injury is an attack on who you are. You need to find who you are again. To survive you must do things differently.
- Everyone tries to latch on to the person they were before because ego gets in the way. You have to let go, experience grief then rebuild yourself using different pieces.

Deborah had formed the Independent Living Center, where the focus was on self-help, consumer control and peer approach. She said that rehab perceives the individual with brain injury as a client to be managed and fixed to fit into society. Instead, her Center was adaptive and inventive. Members would go to participants' homes to make helpful suggestions. For example, one man was going to be put in a home because of problems caused by his poor memory; he would leave the apartment with the stove on and risk fire breaking out. A solution to the problem involved putting a light at the front door which was connected to the stove so that it flashed when the stove was left on.

Later that week, on a sunny afternoon, as squirrels danced through the autumn leaves and sparrows cheekily took grain from between the hooves of the carriage horses, Ted and I walked through Central Park to Mt Sinai Hospital for our most important appointment. Eventually we reached the marble halls of the hospital and were ushered into Dr Gordon's consulting room, feeling honoured that such an eminent person would give us his time.

I had put such an effort into travelling to New York and securing an opportunity to speak to this eminent world expert on brain injury yet I had not thought what questions to ask him! When he asked me 'What can I do for you?' my brain went blank. 'I want the keys that unlock the door to set free the brain-injured person,' I blurted out. I was shaking inside. What a stupid thing to say. We'd travelled halfway around the world and I'd asked such a question. Beside me I could sense Ted groaning inwardly thinking, 'now she's done it!'

To our relief my request was met with a warm smile. He then offered his golden key of advice for recovery:

- Remember that the process of trying to constantly reconcile who you were, who you are and who you want to be will never end.
- Don't give up hope.
- Be relentless.

- Realise that more is being found out about brain injury. The past 15 years research has concentrated on survival for people with brain injury. Scholarship now indicates that there are many health-related issues including endocrine and pituitary dysfunction, body changes, colds, flu, respiratory difficulties, continence problems etc.
- Write everything down.
- Realise there is no golden pill to make you better.
- Never give up.

Dr Gordon then took us on a personal tour of the new Mt Sinai Rehabilitation wing and explained what was being done there. We were most touched by his kindness. As we walked back through Central Park the stars came out in a Prussian blue sky and a half-moon hung above the lit Chrysler Building. It was our last night in the Big Apple and we had found so much encouraging knowledge.

Waiting for breakfast the next morning I picked up a newspaper, the only one I had tried to read during our trip. An article entitled 'Music and strong spirit carry pianist past adversity' caught my attention. Ana Maria Trenchi Bottazzi was to play her 40th concert at Carnegie Hall that night. In 1961 her car had ploughed into a truck on an icy road. A surgeon removed 15 blood clots and replaced her forehead with a platinum plate. But he could not replace her energy, her coordination or her ability to recall pages of music. Those qualities took years of work to re-emerge. Pain initially prevented her from striking a single piano key, but she never believed the surgeon who said she would never perform again. After 13 years of recovering her physical and mental abilities Bottazzi returned to the concert stage with a repertoire of 3,000 pieces played from memory. She was awarded the All Nations' Woman's League Woman of the Year in 1982, a United Nations award as an outstanding person in 1984 and the New York Governor's Outstanding Achiever's Award in 1993.

As our plane soared over New York I could just imagine her music soaring around Carnegie Hall and I thought 'we *can* fly'.

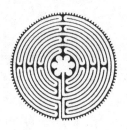

24.
Getting out of the labyrinth through writing, speaking and listening to others with brain injury

Experience is not what happens to a person.
It's what a person does with what happens to them.
Aldous Huxley

2005 Journal
Each morning Lovey and Cloud waddle out of their cage and stumble and shuffle their way to the deck, flap up to the railing to twirl and bob, then squash together in the birdbath where they sit contentedly, enjoying the view from their bathroom. On cold winter days I top up their bath with warm water. When they emerge from their ablutions, their toes are pink, warm and steaming, and their feathers white as snow. After their bath they flutter awkwardly up to the apex of our roof and sit there, like watch-birds of the valley, leaving a white chalky powder on the surface of the water.

Just as Lovey and Cloud daily leave their cage, slowly and gradually I've been able to leave my 'cage of ABI' (acquired brain injury). Fourteen years have now passed since the year my life was broken. Although I still have 'good' and 'bad' days (and weeks), overall I've progressed. It is wonderful that as time goes by I've learnt to work things out so that I can understand more clearly. I think the most important factor helping me put things together in my head was the way my father instilled in me, from early childhood, the belief that I could think things through for myself.

Just as Lovey and Cloud shed white powder from their feathers, I've shed much of my pre-accident life. A couple of years ago, I reluctantly resigned from school because most of my weekly store of energy was consumed by the day and a half I was teaching. I was also speaking to many brain injury support groups. I grudgingly had to admit to myself that I would never achieve my goal of returning to full-time teaching or capture my dream of becoming a school principal. Speaking about brain injury and my book Doing Up Buttons became my priority.

Chasing Ideas

During the decade following my accident I was so fortunate to be able to develop and teach over 4,000 philosophy/thinking workshops with my students. My search for understanding about thinking, both a response to the revelation I had in intensive care and Dad's passion about the importance of thinking well, led me to struggle and stretch my brain, creating attention-grabbing and interesting workshops. In the philosophy/thinking classroom our brains caught fire with ideas as we discussed issues and concepts, laughed, joked and made puns. Visiting teachers remarked that they had never seen students so switched on to ideas, and amazingly, as I switched on my students' brains they switched on my brain. The process of being constantly challenged to figure out new important issues to discuss, and trying to keep up with my student's lightning-fast brains helped me learn how to gain thinking skills as well.

I made notes about our wise and wonderful discussions and wrote another book, *Chasing Ideas* (Finch Publishing and Jessica Kingsley Publishers), which has been translated into Taiwanese, Chinese and Arabic. It seemed extraordinary that it was possible to progress from being someone who could not think (even to find the right words to ask for bread in a shop) to someone who could write a book about thinking, especially a book endorsed by Dr Edward de Bono!

As I chased ideas I re-learnt to think, speak, listen and understand. I was constantly doing 'brain exercises' as I talked with my students. Talking is thinking out loud. I know I rarely spoke in the first years after my accident but once I forced myself to think and talk with my students, and listen carefully to their concepts, I found that I was sorting out my ideas and 'growing' new ideas — making connections in my head.

When I wrote that book I'd hoped that it could be used in rehab programs to help people with brain injury get their brains going again. I believe that putting in an effort to practise thinking and trying to express my thoughts made an incredible difference to my life. I wouldn't be where I am now, if I had not exercised and stretched my brain through chasing ideas. And indeed, now the neuroplasticity of the brain, its ability to adapt and create alternative pathways, is widely discussed and better understood.

By using stories, objects and happenings as symbols of 'big ideas' about important issues such as truth, honesty, ownership, fairness and trust, the 'boredom factor' could be bypassed and the students' curiosity stimulated. If I started a lesson saying, 'Today we are going to discuss the important issue of stealing and ownership' there well might be a massive groan from the class. From there it would be an uphill battle to engage the students with the issues. Instead I set my student's brains on fire by using vomit — combining imagination, humour and enthusiasm I told them a little true story unlock their minds:

> *'Just the other day I was waiting at the doctors' surgery. I was admiring the lovely newly-installed carpet, when in walked a mother and her green-faced son. After sitting down the boy promptly vomited all over the new carpet. I immediately sat up and took notice because I wondered who owned*

> the vomit (who would take responsibility for it). Well, the mum obviously thought the receptionist owned the vomit (or the floor it was on), but in return the receptionist made it plain the mother owned the child and the vomit!'

Once my students started having fun discussing this little story they chased all sorts of ideas and thus thought more broadly and deeply about what it means to own something.

April Fools' Day provided me with a great opportunity to talk about truth and lies. A visit to the zoo opened up ideas about animal rights. Anzac Day provided a prompt for us to discuss all the good, bad and curious things about war. The Olympic Games gave us a chance to discuss sport, fairness and cheating.

To open up discussions I developed what I called 'Handy Thinking'® tools to help the students order their thoughts and approach an issue or problem from many different perspectives.

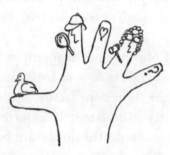

Our thumb reminded us to 'pigeonhole' the idea and ask what other things are similar. Our pointer finger reminded us to point to or find the facts and ask ourselves what are the facts about the issue. Our middle finger (which is in the middle of our hand like our heart is in the middle of our body) reminded us to find the feelings and ask what are the feelings associated with the issue. Our ring finger reminds us of rings. Rings have a hole in them: to look at the whole issue we need to ask ourselves what are the good, bad and curious points. Our little finger reminds us to ask 'What if?', to list actions that could be taken and note the consequences of each action.

Chasing ideas with my students was one of the highlights of my life, but my general health and exhaustion had only marginally improved after 11 years of struggling hard to return to my 'old' life of being a teacher. It was at this time that Handy Thinking helped me take stock of the situation. I made the decision to let go of teaching. I had to face the fact that it would be wiser to use my limited energy to write and speak. Once I was no longer teaching, I could focus on new opportunities and challenges including: speaking with principals, teachers, parents and students at educational conferences, workshops and meetings. Ted pointed out that now I speak to principals, instead of being one!

It was only after 14 years spent engrossed in the mystery of brain injury that another epiphany about the words 'the most important thing you own are your own thoughts' became clear. 'Your own thoughts' are not simply *what* you think (your knowledge, understanding and insight) but it also incorporates *how* you think, that is, your attitude.

Talk About Change

Instead of spending my days thinking up philosophy sessions for my students, I now had a new task. I wanted to put together interesting presentations that would open up people's minds to look at brain injury and how to cope with life's challenges in a fresh way. But most importantly, I wanted to encourage people to never give up hope. I searched for symbols to make the presentations interesting, amusing and entertaining because if there was anything I had learnt from decades of teaching and my own experience, it was that humour, the unexpected and metaphors can open people's minds in a powerful way.

In searching for a way to share some of my revelations about brain injury I used one of Dad's favourite sayings. He loved fishing and he always cultivated his own worms for bait under an old hessian bag in the vegetable garden. When he went fishing he'd collect worms in a jam tin where they'd intertwine into a wriggling pink mess. Dad would say to me 'Chick, when you've got a lot of problems, they get all mixed up like the worms in the can. What you need to do is tip the worms out of the can and untangle them. Then you can tackle them one by one.'

But what if the problems seemed too poisonous to be worms? What if they were more like snakes? I'd then produce a jiggling bag and gingerly pull out a large squirming snake. I developed the knack of making a five foot long rubber snake move in most a realistic way. Much to the horror of the audience I'd fling the snake onto the stage — it certainly made them sit up and take notice! This little act led me to talk about how I'd learnt to turn snakes (things that were hurting me) into ladders (things that helped me escape from the pit of brain injury).

I'd talk about the 'Hate-snake' — how I hated myself but finally learned to treat myself like my own best friend rather than my own worst enemy. To escape from the 'Revenge-snake', when I ruminated about getting revenge on Mr X, I needed myself to forgive him. There was also the 'Mirage-snake' for when I 'saw' things that we not really there. I would explain that I couldn't turn all my snakes into ladders. I couldn't turn my 'Pain-snake' or 'Double-vision-snake' into a ladder, but I have become immune to their poison and we co-habit together.

As well as a rubber snake I used the ingredients of a cake to sum up the brain injury experience. Calling it the 'Coping Cake' I'd assemble flour, sugar, milk and eggs in a mixing bowl and ask the audience to suggest what different ingredients might represent. Ideas would abound and discussions followed. Flour made up the bulk of the cake — what was the most important part of coping? — some people would suggest hope, others adapting. Sugar represented the sweet things in life and audience members shared things they thought helped them, varying from chocolate to nature. Everyone agreed about the need of the milk of human kindness and so forth. Then I'd show the mess in bowl to the audience and asked if this was a cake. Of course the answer was 'No'. Someone would say, 'First you have to beat the mixture, then bake it'.

I'd then produce a giant spoon and explain to professionals that their task was to encourage their client to pick up the spoon, and to put an effort into their own recovery. If the audience was made up of people with brain injury, I'd encourage them to throw themselves wholeheartedly into picking up the spoon and putting an effort into assembling and mixing all the things that could help them to cope with their brain injury.

As a 'take home' message I'd make 'golden spoons' (white plastic teaspoons from the supermarket that I would spray with gold paint) as symbols to remind them to 'pick up the spoon' and put in the effort to tackle their issues to cope with brain injury. People have found ways of coping. When I ask for a show of hands from people who have done something they were told they would never do it's heart-warming to see a sea of hands rise in the air, and observe the look of pleasure and pride on the faces of the people with their hands aloft. Another 'take home' message was 'Hope Stones' — like the stone on the cover of this book. Beautiful, polished river pebbles (purchased from a garden supply outlet) with attached small stars (like I used when I was teaching to reward good work) to remind the audience that we *can* find ways to tackle the hard things (like the hard stone) and reach for the stars.

My daughter Helen often says to me 'Mum, you're always trying to turn a piece of poo into a rose' so sometimes I conclude a talk by giving out roses to encourage people to turn their 'piece of poo into a rose'.

I'll never forget one three day conference put on by a Head Injury Service where I ran workshops. To conclude our time together we completed assembling and discussing the ingredients in the 'Coping Cake', then each person took turns to stir the mixture. Some people had to contend with physical difficulties which made this task difficult, however I'm sure there were many private wishes for 'luck' to help us find new ways of coping as they stirred the mixture. The very large cake was baked and we all enjoyed a slice at our farewell lunch. I'd asked the organisers of the conference if they knew of a nearby source of cut roses so Ted and I could give one to each attendee. We were overwhelmed when the whole group then burst into song with Bette Midler's 'The Rose' while they held their roses. The organisers had secretly taught everyone the song. I don't think there was a dry eye in the hall.

The first edition of *Doing Up Buttons* had been out of print for several years and yet people were still contacting me about the book. Then Harry Troedel, a young man with brain injury rang me to see where he could get a copy for his friends 'so they would understand'. I lent him my last copy and to my surprise he emailed me a couple of days later to say he thought that the book should be reprinted so that it was available to help people. Harry made some phone calls and obtained some funding and I put in enough money for Penguin Books to reprint 1,000 copies. Harry and I gave them away from the Transport Accident Commission's stall at the 5th Congress on Brain Injury in Melbourne in 2005.

This experience was remarkable because I had no clue that the book had been so useful for people with brain injury, their families and professionals. It was wonderful to meet nurses who told me how they had purchased copies of the book to give to their patients and I learnt that the book was a recommended text at universities from Darwin to Perth to Sydney.

As well as giving out the book we also gave attendees at the Congress 'Hope Stones'. Although these stones had been enthusiastically received by audiences after other presentations, Ted was unsure of how professional delegates would react to them. In spite of Ted's apprehensiveness, we ended up giving away 40kg of Hope Stones! People kept coming up to me throughout the conference, patting their pockets and saying 'I've still got it with me'. Since then, when I've encountered some of these people, they still speak about the remembering the message of their Hope Stone.

People with brain injury are constantly reaching for the stars. With humour, and sometimes irony, many have generously shared the discoveries they've made.

Several common themes have emerged over the years. People have often struggled to find information to help them understand their brain injury; they have found comfort knowing they are not alone, and they really want to help others striving to cope. So many people are sad and confused, caught up in the predicaments that brain injury creates. Many times I've been asked: 'Why did this have to happen to me?'; 'Why was I meant to live, was there a reason why I survived, or was I just lucky?'; 'How can I deal with my sadness and hopelessness? I've lost myself and my life!' People have said to me: 'I can't stop crying. I'm so sad'; 'I get so upset all the time'; 'Things seem absolutely dreadful'; ' Sometimes I think I'm crazy'; 'I can't let go of awful thoughts'; 'I can't understand what people say'; 'I feel stupid but I'm not stupid'; 'I hate myself!'; 'I feel like a waste of space'; 'I hate what I've become'; 'I need a "cone of protection" like Maxwell Smart, to keep out my anger'.

Sometimes words were not needed for stories to emerge. At one morning tea in Perth put on by a brain injury support organisation I was greeting people as they came into the hall when I met Molly. Her carer wheeled her into the hall in a horizontal position. Although Molly could not speak, she expressed her thoughts clearly. During my presentation I talked about how guilty I felt for affecting my elderly parents' lives because of my brain injury, when suddenly Molly let out a heartrending cry. Later, watching her face when I was speaking to her, I understood that she also felt guilty because she had affected her parents' life. At times I can still hear the echo of Molly's cry in my head, and I wonder how she is.

With insight and awareness people have also shown they can see the funny side of their experiences. Murray was pleased to explain that sometimes he did strange things when he was frustrated. Once he'd thrown his new computer keyboard in the creek because he was so angry the keys were not in alphabetical order. Jim had been so frustrated, and couldn't communicate his anger and bewilderment, so he'd chased an emu across the paddocks — a dangerous thing to do as emus can attack people with their powerful big feet. John explained that he was placed in a secure locked room in the rehabilitation hospital and he longed to escape back home to the bush.

> *'I just had ta get outta there. For weeks I planned me escape. Then the big day came. I had me pajamas over me clothes, I asked the nurse for somethin' she left the door unlocked, I got out of me room, sneaked down the corridor, squeezed outta a window, crawled through them bushes, ran across the grass till I came to a high wire fence. I stopped and thought to meself "What the #@*$ will I do now? I dunno know where I live, I dunno know how to get there." I just couldn't figure out what ta do next. So I just ran back across the*

grass, crawled through them bushes, squeezed in the window, sneaked down the corridor and got back inta bed.'

John could think and plan some things very well BUT he'd overlooked the most important consideration — where would he go?

A number of people have said 'I'm a better person now. Brain injury has taught me about myself and others'; 'My accident taught me patience'; 'I've got a good sense of humour. At least I've got some sense! People without ABI haven't any sense or a sense of humour!' From my contact with hundreds of people with brain injury in various parts of Australia and overseas I have learnt that there is a very strong bond between people struggling to cope with brain injury.

Atticus put it superbly when he said: 'There's a lot of wisdom in this room full of people with ABI, a lot of experiences'.

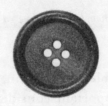

25.
Acquiring Better Insight into the Acquired Brain Injury experience

The great pleasure in life is doing what people say you cannot do.
W. Bagehot

2012 Journal
It's now the 21st anniversary of that fateful day of my accident and it's autumn again. The Japanese maple leaves glow scarlet in the sunshine, the crimson king parrots have departed after their 'pit stop' for breakfast and I've fed the cockatoos. This autumn I am celebrating being alive plus I've just ceased being a university student and returned to my usual occupation of being a student of life. Now I can add Dr to my name. I almost have to pinch myself to make sure I am not dreaming. Each day I am so thankful that I did not die in the accident, or by my own hand afterwards.

Four years ago I found myself searching for more 'string'. This time I was looking for something worthwhile to do to use my understanding about brain injury, teaching and talking about change. Yet I was at a loss about what new direction to take on my journey of life.

One day, when I'd completed my 'Talk About Change' presentation at a conference for Disability Liaison Officers from universities and was chatting over coffee, two different people suggested that I should use my experience and knowledge to complete a PhD. In doing this I could use my knowledge and information to help people understand and gain better insight into brain injury. Although I had put such a tremendous effort into regaining my life and finding a way out of the labyrinth of brain injury I still experienced many brain injury and accident related difficulties. Although I had started to think I could now move on from a life dominated by brain injury, speaking to these women reminded me that perhaps I could still find out important information and have greater opportunity to speak to professionals on behalf of people with brain injury who could not speak for themselves.

However, I thought I could never do the research required and write a 100,000-word PhD with my troublesome double vision, limited memory, constant pain, and fatigue (I still need an afternoon nap) and my one finger typing. Then I heard about doing a PhD by exegesis — by project — with a 40,000-word thesis. Hmmm. What a curious thought. Now I just *might* be able to devise a project, like I had devised curriculum at school. The following week I heard about the philosophy of phenomenology where a researcher looks at issues from the point of view of the participant as they reflect upon their experience. The combination of the concepts of exegesis and phenomenology fired my imagination and led me to a new challenge.

I explored the possibilities, attended one university information evening and spoke with one lecturer, Dr Paul Ramcharan, who subsequently became my supervisor. It was serendipitous that I spoke at that Disability Liaison Officers' conference, otherwise I wouldn't have embarked on a PhD. Talk about a mature aged student — I'm now 68!) Thus I started on a learning journey that was to consume four years of my life, and result in a traditional PhD of 100,000 words.

By approaching brain injury from the perspective of the 'insider', the person with brain injury, I set out to find a way that would support, encourage and empower participants to reflect upon factors that influenced their life negatively and to find a way to address these issues. Most importantly I wanted to find factors that positively affected their wellbeing so that this information could be passed on. The objective of the study was to devise a 'tool', based on education and learning principles, to gather information that could be used as a learning resource to help people with brain injury to feel and fare better. The study also aimed to help carers understand and cope better and to give professionals a new way to talk about brain injury, so they could better help their clients.

All those years ago in New York, when I visited Dr Gordon at Mt. Sinai Hospital, I had been like John who tried to escape from the rehab hospital only to realise he didn't know where he lived. I'd put such an effort into getting to see Dr Gordon that when he asked me 'What can I do for you?' I didn't know what to say — I hadn't planned that far! I simply blurted out 'I want the golden keys that unlock the door to set free the brain injured person'. My PhD was a continuation of this search for the 'golden keys'.

At this time I was also talking at conferences to health professionals and constantly searching for different ways to engage people in considering brain injury in fresh ways. I sometimes used the old nursery rhyme about Jack and Jill to introduce the subject. Jack and Jill went up the hill to fetch a pail of water. When Jack fell down he broke his crown so he went to bed to mend his head with vinegar and brown paper. Yet it takes a lot more than vinegar and brown paper to mend broken heads (and hearts, lives and dreams). My study was an attempt to find something better than vinegar and brown paper.

The origins of this nursery rhyme are really fascinating. It was literally about 'losing your head'. 'Jack' stood for King Louis

XVI of France and Jill, (who came tumbling after), represented Marie Antoinette. Apparently back in the eighteenth century it was believed that after your head had been severed, consciousness remained for eight seconds. How often have we seen pictures of a severed head being held aloft by the hair? This custom showed the head to the crowd, but also allowed the eyes in the head to gaze at their own body. This is yet another interesting metaphor for brain injury — you lose your head. You can still see your body but in some strange way your head is disconnected and no longer has control over your body.

I often used this metaphor when I was speaking to health professionals. I wanted them to see brain injury from another perspective. Instead of using the rubber snake to grab their attention, when I said the words 'they held the severed head aloft...' I would hold up high what looked like, for a split second, a real head. Actually it was only an old pink rubber ball with a 'wig' of black knitting wool attached to a bit of contact adhesive plastic which was stuck on the ball with a loop of masking tape. As some people in the audience let out a gasp I could rip the 'wig' off the ball and bounce it, explaining that in the same way as people can mistake a ball and some wool for a head it is possible to mistake people with brain injury, and not see the *real* person hiding within the brain injured person.

My study was my attempt to find a way to help re-connect the head and body. In order to re-connect and recapture our lives following brain injury we need to accept our situation, focus on our difficulties and devise coping strategies. Instead I found that research indicated that as people reflected on their losses and difficulties they became depressed. Hardly surprising! So my challenge was to find a way to help people with brain injury understand more about their condition and reflect on their experience in a positive way as well as finding out what information would be helpful for them.

As well as making wigs and talks I was making progress researching academic papers and brain injury support websites and writing about what the studies identified regarding brain injury. There was so much information and a lot of the research didn't appear to be very positive. The majority of studies involved tests and questionnaires, and focused on what the professionals, working within certain areas, identified as important. These included areas such as loss of IQ, memory, and self-awareness after brain injury; depression and suicide, fatigue, pain, and post-traumatic stress.

Reviewing the studies, I saw that there had been so much effort, expertise and money spent researching different 'bits' of the person. Yet these studies did not look at the person as a whole. I was reminded of John Godfry Saxe's poem about the blind men and the elephant.

It was six men of Indostan
To learning much inclined,
Who went to see the Elephant
(Though all of them were blind),
That each by observation
Might satisfy his mind.

The First approached the Elephant,
And happening to fall
Against his broad and sturdy side,
At once began to bawl:
'God bless me! But the Elephant is very like a wall!'
'...like a spear!' '...like a snake!' '...like a tree!' '...like a fan!'

So oft in theologic wars,
The disputants, I ween,
Rail on in utter ignorance
Of what each other mean,
And prate about an Elephant
Not one of them has seen.

(The Blind Men and the Elephant: John Godfry Saxe 1816–87)

I decided that I did not want to look at a specific 'bit' of the person with brain injury, instead I did want to find out how brain injury affected the *whole* person. To do this I needed to hear how people perceived their everyday experiences and about the issues that affected their 'lifeworld' as they saw it. So I scribbled this little ditty based on Saxe's poem.

The outside of an Elephant
Is made up of different parts
But that's not all Elephant is, Elephant has mind and heart.
Elephant's more than leg and trunk and hide and eyes and meat.
Elephant's more than tail and ears and side and tusk and feet.

In circus, zoo, and forest too
Elephant works in fields and more
A family pet, a faithful friend,
He can run amok and gore.
Carrying tourists, logs or heavy loads, his attributes are many
But rogue and wild, and strong and huge, Elephant's very scary!

Why, oh why, I ask you,
Does this massive wrinkly beast
Disobey his master
Or sit upon a seat?
He sways and dances (it is true) when tethered to a stake
When looking into all of this, of sense we cannot make.

The essence of the Elephant
Is mighty hard to find
It's not locked up in books or film
Or held in someone's mind.
If only Elephant could speak, and tell us what he knows
Then, and only then, could we discover how he goes.

Searching for an interesting, non-medical, fun, non-threatening way to help participants to focus on their experience and tell me how they get by or cope with their challenges in a completely different way was a challenge.

Brain injury is complicated, difficulties people with brain injury experience are complicated, how people cope with brain injury is complicated, and it was complicated developing a non-judgmental 'tool' to help people reflect on their experience. Helping people with brain injury to remember factors that negatively and positively affect their lives is an example of what Salman Rushdie calls a P2C2E (a Process too Complicated to Explain)!

In my office I still had the fancy bird cage in which I'd take my doves Lovey Dovey and Cloud to television interviews after the first edition of *Doing Up Buttons* was published. The birds reminded me to discuss how I felt I wasn't a 'proper' person, just like fantail doves weren't 'proper' birds. I'd often looked at the cage and thought of brain injury as just like being locked in a cage when the key is thrown away. In my search for an engaging, original, non-medical, non-threatening way to connect and communicate with people with brain injury, I found myself drawn to the metaphor of how brain injury 'imprisons' the person.

So I decided to use the cage, my old walking stick and a pole with a flying pig on the top to hold what I called 'Talk-about cards'. These cards had things written on them that people with brain injury had talked to me about over the years. I called this metaphor for brain injury 'Keys to the ABI Cage'. As well as being a metaphor for brain injury it also provided a guide to help participants with memory, cognitive and physical difficulties reflect on their experience in a completely different and positive way. The tool divided the complicated issues and consequences of brain injury into three main themes and this simplification allowed participants to reflect on their own experience.

Keys to the ABI cage

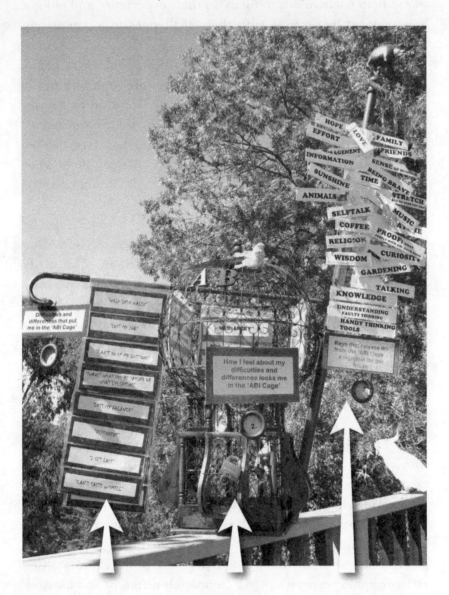

1. Our difficulties and differences can put us in the ABI cage.

2. How we feel about our differences and difficulties can lock us in the ABI cage.

3. Keys that can release us from the ABI cage.

To create my 'Keys to the ABI Cage' I inserted my old walking stick horizontally into the bird cage. Hanging on it was a sign that said 'Our differences and difficulties can PUT us in the ABI Cage' and a number of talk-about cards (including things such as 'I forget my name', 'I can't walk properly', 'I get lost', 'I fall over' — all expressing the difficulties of brain injury).

Then on the front of the cage, near a shiny brass padlock, was a sign that read 'How we feel about our differences and difficulties can LOCK us in the ABI Cage'. Talk-about cards were locked inside the cage (How we can feel: sad, disappointed, distressed, depressed, mad, angry, frustrated and crazy, bad, guilty, and so forth). There were also objects that were symbols of how we might feel with brain injury. A crushed soft drink can really resonated with many of the participants who asked me to unlock the cage so they could take out the can. 'This is my life' they would say as they held the can.

Tied to the right side of the cage was a long wooden pole topped by a flying pig (yes pigs can fly and the impossible can happen) and the sign 'Keys can RELEASE us from the ABI Cage'. The pole was covered with a large selection of Talk-about cards naming things that can help us feel better: 'sunshine', 'my family', 'information', 'time' etc. Tiny objects such as a miniature sun, a tiny wedding ring, a mini book, a minute clock, a watering can, a tiny dog were attached to the talk-about cards.

Brain injury support organisations ran information about my project in their newsletters and I had dozens of phone conversations with people who wanted to participate in the study. It was quite a complicated process: talking to people on the phone to make sure they fitted the criteria (which included being two years post-injury and not going through a bad patch and feeling fragile); making and sending out the Reflection kit (a digital device with a Power Point™ presentation with a voice over and sheets to fill in); posting explanatory letters and consent forms; making interview appointments; packing up the cage; driving to interviews within two hours of our home;

contacting people afterwards to see if they were okay and not upset after reflecting on their experience; and sending out thank you cards. My one track mind found juggling all of this at once rather tricky!

We arranged to meet wherever the individual person felt comfortable: coffee shops, libraries and so forth. When we get together I'd introduce the participants to the bird cage which Ted and I would set up, then I'd show them an explanation in a Power Point™ presentation so that they became familiar with things we'd be discussing. Then I'd hand them *another* set of talk-about cards and place a 'Do' and 'Don't' box on the table. They simply placed each card in a box and talked about the issue *if they wanted to*. They were in control of the interview, there were no questionnaires to fill out, or tests to complete. I simply asked people to talk about the words on the card they were holding or whatever the words reminded them about.

I was concerned that reflecting on such experiences could be upsetting. So my focus became things that helped people or 'Keys'. Participants were encouraged help other people with brain injury by sharing 'keys' that might open the 'ABI Cage' for them. What a privilege it was to have 36 people with brain injury (I intended to interview 30 people, but I still have difficulty counting!), five people who care for and support family members with brain injury (I was careful not to refer to them as 'carers' because if you need a 'carer' you can feel a lesser person) and five professionals, generously allow me into their world, to see and feel their experiences and learn from their wisdom.

Ted and the entire family (including our seven grandchildren) surrounded me with unconditional encouragement and interest. Ted supported me each step of the long journey, drove me to each interview, set up the computer and sound recording equipment, and assisted in carrying and setting up the large bird cage.

The cage was cumbersome and awkward and provided some

unpredictable, dicey moments. Manhandling it to a television station for an interview, Ted bent over and split some stitches from recent minor surgery in his back. He asked me to look to see if it was okay. I peeked beneath his jacket and saw that his shirt was soaked with blood. 'It's OK Darling' I fibbed. Somehow I managed to focus on the interview and, as soon as it was over, we rang the surgeon who fortunately restitched the wound immediately!

I often think of the various people who shared their experiences with humility, respect and admiration. They were so eager to communicate in the hope they could help other people cope with brain injury. They displayed such courage, wisdom, determination and kindness. I'm so pleased that my 'Keys to the ABI Cage' helped many to see and understand more. My birdcage helped Ben (who'd spent seven years denying that he had brain injury) accept that yes, he did have brain injury. William said 'The cage has let me open up my eyes'. Liam thought that the cage 'has helped me come to terms with things ...I sort of sat down and thought about things' and Sally remarked 'Now I understand. Medical terms are hard enough if you don't have brain injury, but if you do, it's like another language.'

Completing my PhD was an exciting project. It revealed greater insight into what people with brain injury want. Now I can start putting together a different sort of learning resource — developed from people with brain injury for people with brain injury. Based on my own experience and the interviews I conducted I believe beyond doubt that people with brain injury have an enormous capacity to help themselves, beyond what medical help can achieve. I believe that they can identify their issues and find individual ways forward and help themselves feel and fare better. They can learn to make some sense of brain injury in knowing that others also experience similar challenges.

A learning resource and a book explaining brain injury to children are next on my list of challenges. Once I have finished writing maybe I can focus on things other than brain injury!

From personal experience and from hearing from others with brain injury I believe that HOPE is a key to unlock our brains. I think that HOPE stands for Help Other Possibilities Emerge. Hope helps us find a way through the labyrinth of acquired brain injury.

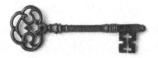

26.
Keys to the ABI Cage

So what did I discover in my four years of study? As I analysed the transcripts from the interviews I was looking for 'blind spots' or areas generally not the focus of academic studies, the things that negatively or positively affected the person as they took on the challenge of trying to 'get by' or cope with a 'new' life — a life changed by brain injury. Addressing these issues is important for everyone dealing with people with brain injury while also having implications for new and experienced health professionals in both their day-to-day contact with clients and their research.

My study demonstrated that brain injury not only damages the person's brain, body and beliefs, it also damages their hope, honour, trust, safety and security. The person mourns the loss of their 'old' self and life, their loss of understanding, their loss of trust of themselves (to do or say the 'right' thing) and their loss of trust in other people (who judge them as fake, dumb, drunk etc). Some people feel they can't trust the 'experts', that their experience is the result of fate, God, or luck, or some kind of punishment. Some people feel ashamed 'because they are not like a normal person', they can't understand or communicate normally and they can't control their emotions. People with brain injury are damaged by the emotional fallout of their injury. They feel sad (disappointed, depressed and distressed), mad (angry, frustrated and crazy) and bad (guilty, stupid and embarrassed).

A great deal of academic literature asserts that people with brain injury lack self-awareness. However by using the bird cage and cards people showed they did have awareness of many of their problems. Nevertheless they often hid their difficulties because of shame, or because they thought the listener would not understand or be empathetic. Keys to the ABI Cage was developed as a tool to help people to reflect on their ABI experience in a constructive way, to express their self-awareness.

In developing the tool I employed many learning theories about how motivation, engagement and perceptions of success can affect the learner, how people are strongly motivated to preserve their self-worth (they don't want people to think they are stupid) and everyone can experience success in sharing insights into brain injury because there are no right or wrong answers. I also used the theory of 'flow' wherein people understand the goals and thus become absorbed in unpacking issues. The cage used what's called 'active learning' where people are actively engaged in the process and participants can use their own preferred learning style. The cage also made use of the theory of association: words, pictures and symbols. The theory of multiple intelligences was also built into the method. Keys to the ABI Cage encouraged and supported people to tell their stories.

The stories people told revealed that they were aware of their many difficulties and how the 'new me' was different to the 'old me'. Keys to the ABI Cage helped them to better understand themselves, to gain greater self-awareness and to think about things that helped them to feel better.

Participants in my PhD study reinforced to me the staggering complexity of brain injury. Almost all the participants with ABI had been involved in rehabilitation to help limit the effect of damage to brain and body. However although the damage to their beliefs, hope, honour, trust, security and safety greatly affected the way they saw themselves, and, in turn, how they engaged in rehabilitation, it was never a focus of their rehabilitation experience.

Weighing up the plethora of complicated difficulties participants with ABI experience in their day-to-day lives it appears impossible that anything could balance the scales so that life could be tolerable. However, some participants with ABI have found that the negative factors of physical, cognitive, and emotional difficulties and deficits of ABI can be balanced by the positive influences of hope, love, understanding, and learning to work things out for themselves. These are the key things that give life meaning and purpose.

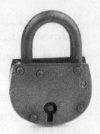

27.
Issues that locked people in the ABI Cage

 1. Loss, lost and trapped

'I am not the person I would have been if I hadn't had the accident.'

'I wish I could have one more day without a brain injury just to be the person that died once more — to be with my family the way I used to.'

'[I feel] the frustration of not knowing who I am, and the lack of understanding of brain injury.'

'I compare myself to my family/friends/peers/workmates; to what I want to do with my life and what I am capable of.'

'I'm frightened because I can't trust myself and I can't trust other people and I can't trust health professionals.'

'When I don't understand what people are saying I feel frustrated... embarrassed.'

'I walked outside and never came back — what else might happen?'

People with brain injury are overwhelmed not only by physical, mental, communication and emotional difficulties and pain, they are also overpowered by a sense of loss, of being a 'different' person. They are aware that they have lost the 'old self' and are struggling to live with their 'new selves'. Some participants spoke of the sadness of realising and accepting that they would never be their 'old self' again.

LOST THE 'OLD' ME

Participants demonstrated they did have self-awareness by telling stories about how they constantly compared their 'old' and 'new' self, and how they thought people (including family, friends, health and legal professionals) could be more understanding and treat them with greater kindness. Many stories demonstrated that life prior to their ABI seemed 'more fair' than their post-ABI life, where they had no choice and little power. They felt bewildered and confused because they could not make sense of, or understand what people were saying, what they should do, or how they should accomplish simple tasks.

CAN'T TRUST MY 'NEW SELF'

The multiple losses people suffered compounded the feeling that the 'old self' that they knew, understood, trusted and depended on had gone and the 'new self' could not be controlled, trusted or understood. They felt cut off and isolated from normal people. They felt bewildered and could not understand the 'new self', the 'stranger' who had taken over their body, brain and life. Just getting by was complicated, tricky, and demanded all their attention and effort. This 'new self' could not be depended on; for example, they could do some things on one day but not the next, at one time of day but not at another time.

They could no longer trust themselves; they were aware that they did and said the wrong thing and, as a consequence, lost confidence in themselves. They were aware they could not control their tongue; they were sometimes not tactful and their decisions were not right.

CAN'T TRUST OTHERS
Almost every participant told of experiences that proved that they could not trust other people. Most spoke of 'disappointing' encounters, when they thought people would understand/have empathy and sympathy for the difficulties they were experiencing. When other people didn't understand (and make allowances) participants became more wary of trusting.

MY FAMILY AND FRIENDS DON'T UNDERSTAND
One third of the people interviewed expressed disappointment with the way their family didn't understand, some felt 'scared' and had 'lost trust' in their families. Fred was 'physically attacked... smacked by my wife', while Melissa was distressed because her parents would accuse her of being lazy when she was trying hard and suffered from 'bad fatigue'. A majority of participants had lost trust in their friends who did not 'see what was really going on', or who said they seemed to be 'OK'. Pete said he wished he could reply, 'Oh yeah. Swap places with you then'.

Many people expressed distress that they did not receive enough care or understanding from medical professionals. Their stories inferred that they thought professionals would be the one group of people who would understand them. A large number of participants were distressed because of the pessimistic outcomes suggested by professionals.

GUILT
A number of participants doubted themselves. They said they felt guilty and asked if I thought they were an 'imposter'. Many stated that they wished they were more damaged with broken limbs so people would understand they were 'injured' or 'damaged'.

STIGMA
The people I interviewed were generally confused and frustrated with their changed life and told stories that illustrated the stigma of ABI. They felt exposed and vulnerable so they tried to hide

their difficulties/differences/deficits from their family, friends, the public and medical professionals.

LOST THEIR TRUST IN GOD AND THE FUTURE

My study revealed that religious beliefs had both a negative and positive impact on participants' lives. Some had lost trust in God and many were struggling to make sense of why God appeared to be punishing them, they queried whether God had caused their ABI to teach them a lesson, or even if they could trust God to protect them the future.

Others said they could no longer trust luck or the future and over half the participants said that they were terrified they would have another accident; if it had happened once, it could happen again. They were afraid that they wouldn't have 'the will or the energy to fight brain injury when it happens again'.

2. No longer like a 'normal' person

'If I was granted a wish today, it wouldn't be to have my sight back. It would be "can I have my left side back" to make me whole again.'

'My hands didn't work properly.'

'I forgot to eat. I didn't have any appetite; I didn't know when I was hungry and when I wasn't.'

'I have a great deal of trouble enunciating words — people find it hard to understand me.'

'It's weird telling you...because you understand what I'm talking about... But then you forget that you couldn't remember to use the phone, so you couldn't actually get any help anywhere, because you couldn't remember what you couldn't remember. I think, looking back now, I thought there was something really, really bad, wrong, and that I'd better not tell anyone. No, not that I shouldn't tell anyone, but that I was embarrassed, ashamed...I don't know, I think I was terrified.'

None of the participants referred to themselves as disabled.

However, they told stories in which they compared themselves to 'normal' people and this comparison had a negative effect on their life. Their difficulties not only made life difficult, they were also symbols that they were not 'normal' any more. They could not function 'normally' in order to do a range of normal things such as walking, driving, working, going out, socialising or travelling; most had balance problems. Some accepted their physical difficulties in a matter-of-fact way, others joked about them, while others ignored their difficulties. Several participants stoically accepted impaired vision, loss of one eye or being legally blind.

It also emerged from many stories that people were struggling with a variety of perplexing 'invisible' issues including 'left neglect' (where they neglected the left side of their body) and distorted vision. A small number of participants spoke about weird metaphysical issues, where they did not know who was talking (the other person or themselves). These invisible issues had a profound effect on their life.

Distorted vision, double vision, and seeing in other peculiar ways affected some participants. If vision was 'confused' it was 'confusing' to see things that were not there — if they couldn't believe their eyes to tell them what was real how did they know what was real? Tunnel vision meant many blind spots and this caused frustration and walking difficulties. People spoke of sometimes 'sensing' someone was in their blind spot, which was disconcerting. These strange and weird aspects of ABI all had a negative effect on the participants' life.

SLEEPING DIFFICULTIES AND EXHAUSTION
Sleeping was a problem for many people, they had difficulty sleeping at night or as one participant expressed it, her brain 'could no longer go to the place of sleep'. However, most adapted to their low energy or fatigue. They accepted that coping with fatigue was part of their life with ABI; they realised they would tire, and learnt to adapt their daily activities to cope with the

mental, physical and emotional exhaustion and weariness.

COMMUNICATION DIFFICULTIES

Many participants spoke of frustration, embarrassment and distress because they couldn't understand what people were saying, and people couldn't understand them. Several participants discussed their puzzling inability to use the telephone, that they did not remember how to do things or 'have the words to ask for help' at an appropriate time. This made them doubt themselves and was taken as proof that they were not normal. Difficulty communicating made them embarrassed, ashamed and afraid they were crazy.

3. Grappling with emotional fallout

'Probably mad/frustrated — that's brain injury in a nutshell.'

'Disappointed is an interesting word, it's too mild for what I felt. I was probably disappointed with myself, disappointed with the doctors, and disappointed with everyone and everything for a while. Um, sad, distressed, and absolute abject despair and futility.'

'I'm so disappointed with life — my illness wasn't my fault.'

'I was depressed and I was powerless.'

'I was very angry, I had terrible anger.'

'Oh God I was really frustrated.'

'It drives you to distraction...trying to make your brain work.'

'Feeling am I going mad? I think I am going mad.'

'I thought I was mad and everyone else was mad.'

'I feel guilty because I can't trust myself — I'm not dependable — with good and bad days my thinking works in stops and starts.'

'They say 'Put the thing over there' and I don't understand — I'm lost.'

'I have not cried since the accident — I feel like I need to cry to get it out you know — I'd love to cry — I have so much to cry about.'

'I went sort of the opposite, I just found everything hilarious. I was really

extreme. I'd sit there and just laugh at everything. Well, I couldn't help myself.'

'I feel like I'm an imposter — I haven't got it all together and things eat away at me — if I tried a bit harder I'd fix myself.'

'I feel bad because people say things that I don't understand and I feel bad. Is it me or maybe the ABI just brought that out?'

'I feel bad because I'm slow and I can't concentrate, I can't understand things.'

SAD, MAD AND BAD

All the people I interviewed identified with the 'sad', 'mad' and 'bad' talk-about cards that were positioned inside the ABI cage. Many expressed that they were disappointed with themselves and their lives, disappointed because they could now no longer achieve their dreams, disappointed because day-to-day survival was difficult, disappointed that their future was changed for the worse financially, and disappointed that they no longer had careers they had loved, disappointed in marriages that had broken down, and disappointed that life was no longer predictable or controllable.

They talked about feeling depressed, hating themselves, having contemplated suicide or disappearing, and feeling powerless. One participant spoke about the reluctance of professionals, family and friends to discuss their suicidal feelings with them. Many participants also identified with the distressed talk-about card — that the ABI experience was distressing.

Anger was a big problem and many people told stories of their terrible anger and rage. However, the majority of respondents reported they had feelings of frustration, they felt annoyance rather than anger — frustration at themselves, at situations they were put in because of having ABI and their loss of choice. All of the participants placed the 'Frustration' talk-about card in the 'Do' box and their stories told of the struggle of trying to cope with a brain and body that does not obey.

Many participants said that in the years following their accident they had believed they had gone mad or insane, that they had frequently questioned if they were crazy. Some thought that everyone else was mad. All were profoundly affected by believing they were insane.

Most participants expressed guilt, either about pain they were causing their family who they felt they had 'let down', or for what they had put their family through. They felt guilty because they had not avoided the accident, because they couldn't make themselves better, or because they had 'let' their ABI affect their life too much. Over half the people interviewed felt guilty they had not 'tried hard enough to make themselves better'.

Many of the male participants expressed feeling like a 'bloody idiot' when they did or said the wrong thing, when their poor balance meant they were unsteady when they walked and so they were accused of being drunk, stereotyped as being a loser, or were declined entry to bars.

The women felt bad about other issues such as doing and saying the wrong thing; one participant elegantly called this the 'loss of social graces'; others queried if the inappropriate action was due to their ABI or because they are 'just stupid?' Not being able to complete simple tasks such as doing up their buttons resulted in them 'feeling pretty stupid actually', being embarrassed because they were 'slow and can't concentrate, or can't understand things'. Over all the people I interviewed were ashamed, afraid and isolated as a result of their emotional fallout.

4. The rehab experience didn't suit me

I'm so angry at the way I was treated — all professionals, even alternative ones are arrogant.'

'In rehab I felt like a meal ticket.'

'I wanted it to be about me. Well, all our problems were different. And I don't like group therapy.'

'Some of those experts that I saw…didn't inspire … they made it harder.'

'Rehab was a waste of time.'

'Rehab was like being in jail — I was a copper.'

'I had to do rehab — I didn't want to do rehab — but you've got to do what you've got to do.'

'My OT was hopeless — it just didn't fit with what I felt I needed.'

'We want to educate the professionals.'

'They don't know what it's like to actually experience the system.'

'I thought they didn't know what they were talking about.'

'The OT kept telling me I wasn't trying enough. It made me mad.'

'They thought I was slow — I was now deaf — what terrible mistake to make!'

'Perhaps the professionals could treat us less like text book cases and consider us as human beings with thoughts and feelings…we are not babies and do not need to be treated like we are.'

'People in rehab were blind to our ability.'

'I felt it was suggested I was lazy, or my motivation damaged.'

'I was told all through my rehab and from other doctors, that the brain will only heal in the first two years, and after that there's not much healing that happens.'

I did not intend to focus upon the rehabilitation experience. Indeed, among over 60 talk-about cards there was only one that said 'Rehab' but this card prompted such a great deal of comment. Some participants spoke about the wonderful, doctor, neuropsychologist or physiotherapist who had made such a difference to their life. Unfortunately, however, over half the people with brain injury interviewed expressed the opinion that the rehabilitation experience had been very upsetting. They felt they had been damaged twice — once by their brain injury and then again by their rehab experience.

The general perception was that during their time in rehab they were not understood, that they had no power, that they were not respected, that they were constantly judged, that they were compelled to complete numerous tests, that they believed their truthfulness was questioned, and that they felt things 'weren't fair'. Many people admitted that they had not been really engaged, that they just wanted their brain injury to go away. The perception was that they were simply a 'meal ticket' for the rehab professionals, or that they believed they were not a 'text book' case although they were treated like one, and thus they felt that the professionals did not really understand. These perceptions had a profound long-term ramifications for their wellbeing.

Some participants had forgotten what was said and done in rehabilitation but not how rehabilitation made them feel. They talked about people and events they did not want to think about, but found they could not forget.

The majority of people I interviewed were informed that the brain heals for up to two years, then the person 'plateaus out'. For many, this two year rule took away their hope.

The statements made by all the people with ABI I interviewed demonstrate that they had awareness and insight of many things that negatively affected their life. Many of them were swamped by their experience, although some had moved from feeling that life was not worthwhile to feeling that life was worthwhile, and a few felt enriched by their struggle.

ABI is complicated, always challenging, and has a catastrophic impact on a person's life and wellbeing.

In retrospect, we've realised the things listed below are dark places in the labyrinth

...*information in medical language is difficult to understand or apply*

...*the term 'mild ABI' is deceptive and doesn't cover how difficult life can be*

...*professionals need to cease putting the 2 or 5 year time limitation on recovery from ABI*

...rehab also needs to focus upon the emotional wellbeing of the person

...people with ABI need to be encouraged and empowered in rehab to find ways to help themselves

...feeling bad because you don't understand the atmosphere or tone of situations.

...struggling to try to understand what is obvious to others.

...rolling lots of problems together so they get tangled and unsolvable.

...unintentionally hurting people.

...not understanding that there are many 'models' or ways of looking at brain injury: the charity model, the medical model, the social model — these can affect how we are treated.

...pushing so hard for what we want that we don't see or value what we have.

...holding onto dammed up feelings.

...trying to work out what to fight for and what to compromise on.

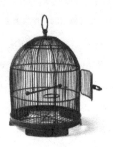

28.
Things that released people from the ABI Cage

Never, never, never, never, never ever give up!

The emotions and perceptions that locked participants in the ABI Cage were just as limiting (if not more so) than their actual brain injury. The most exciting finding from my study was that participants themselves identified a large number of things that could work as 'keys' to unlock the ABI Cage, and give them some control in the healing of body and spirit as well as the creation of a 'new' sense of self. These 'keys' can be used by people with brain injury, their family and friends, professionals in healthcare and the general public.

Key 1: **Hope**

'Um, I guess I don't use the word hope, I just think of it as bloody mindedness. Sheer determination, where I'm mad as hell and I'm not going to take this anymore.'

'I wasn't willing to accept that I would be in a wheelchair in a nursing home for the rest of my life.'

'Hang on; I'm not going to let this beat me!'

'The doctor was quite adamant that after two years you've reached your peak — it took away all my hope — I was frustrated because I thought I was going to get better…but then I thought I'm going to improve…'

Hope is the most important factor that helps people with ABI move forward and find ways to help themselves to feel and fare better. Having hope made them try hard to recapture a worthwhile life, and to be fully involved in making progress.

Hope comes in many guises, from determination to what I call 'wishful thinking'. Sometimes hope comes in the form of refusing to accept the considered opinions of professionals. People who refused to accept the predictions (that they would never walk again, that they would spend their life in a nursing home or in a wheelchair, or that they could not have children), managed to find a way for the impossible to happen. A majority of the people I interviewed had been informed by one professional or another that progress would cease or slow down after the first two or five years. However they all found life in fact continued to improve.

Some people chose to believe that God had spared their life for a reason, some believed in the power of nature and some saw symbols that indicated they were on the right path.

Key 2: **Love**

'Love is extremely important. I believe that if I didn't have my family and husband to come home to, I wouldn't have worked so hard. I don't think I did it for me, I did it so they could have a life.'

'The love and understanding of my oldest and very dear friends and their ongoing support.'

'I think if I didn't have my three cats who loved me unconditionally, to talk to, I wouldn't cope at all.'

'Animals. I have lots — the cats are great, really affectionate.'

> '*Taking responsibility and caring for something else (my animals) — I think it is very big.*'
>
> '*My cats saved my life. I would have "disappeared" but for my cats.*'

Love is of prime importance in empowering and encouraging people to put an effort into finding ways to feel and fare better. Many people I interviewed spoke about how they were loved, supported and sheltered by their family, and how their love for their family also caused them to work harder for their family's sake. In contrast, some participants did not identify love as a 'key'. Instead, they told stories of how they were divorced or estranged from their family through misunderstanding or lack of understanding.

For many people with ABI animals are important. Several participants stated that they would have killed themselves but for their love of their animals. These animals provided the unconditional love these people needed to survive, they felt loved and understood, and this love gave their life meaning.

Other people find love in things they love doing, things that gave them satisfaction and a purpose. It was evident during the interviews in the way people perked up and became enthusiastic that these were more than a diversion — people who are fully engaged with their 'passion' experience love. A huge range of passions were identified: painting, fishing, knitting, going to live shows, gardening, exercise, the gym, writing, and going out for coffee or lunch.

The majority of people I interviewed loved helping others, being useful, having a purpose — particularly when it meant they could help other people with brain injury. Being a volunteer was often an important element in their life as it allowed them to use their sense of empathy and their skills in a meaningful way. Participants in the study connected with the people they were helping and they spoke with pride about their volunteering.

Key 3: **Learning to understand ABI and working things out**

'Gain as much knowledge as you can about your brain injury to help you understand.'

'It was important to understanding my condition.'

'If I'd had the 'Keys to the ABI Cage' earlier on it would have helped me to understand that I wasn't going mad. And it certainly would have given me another way of approaching things too. And perhaps to even ask more questions. Because if I knew that was the situation, then I could relate that to other areas.'

Learning to understand is at the heart of this book, indeed, it is a reason it has been written. It is vital that brain injury is explained clearly, in everyday (not medical) language so that people can make sense of their difficulties, feel empowered to make choices and do things to help themselves. All the participants I interviewed spoke about wanting more information they could understand.

For most people, learning to understand and working things out involved making discoveries about themselves: their self-belief, their attitude of not giving up, of trying to remain positive, and their sense of humour. These traits helped them to be motivated to put in the huge effort required to teach their body to work again, to participate and take advantage of rehabilitation exercises. Many participants also spoke about the importance of finding out what other people with brain injury have done and the value of peer support, how support organisations and writing groups helped them share ideas, learn new skills and express themselves.

People told me about the range of strategies through which they worked things out, for example: patience, minimal stress, simplicity, routine/organisation, structured living, quiet, a healthy diet, exercise, concentration, and tracking progress and achievements.

Key 4: **Learning to face the facts (acceptance)**

'Coming to terms with the fact that I'm not the same person anymore.'

'Redefining who I am and where I want to head to.'

'Admitting to myself I have shortcomings (short-term memory) and learning to employ strategies to assist me with coping with these shortcomings.'

'I now view the world from a changed perspective.'

'Recognising positive things from ABI experience.'

'I have a much greater understanding of life and people.'

'Learning to appreciate life.'

'Looking at every part of my life post the brain bleed as a bonus.'

'Saying I can do something.'

Overwhelmingly I found that people wanted to pass on to others with ABI these important ideas. Many participants commented that they had never had the opportunity to discuss these things, to try to make sense of how they have 'survived' ABI, until they discussed their experience using 'Keys to the ABI Cage'. The cage demonstrated the importance of accepting, self-belief, not giving up, having a positive attitude and a sense of humour. These factors were important for motivation, engagement with others, risk-taking and learning.

Key 5: **Making progress — brain injury is not all bad**

'Being able to talk to people and realise that I am still a "normal" person.'

'Knowing I am making a worthwhile contribution at work.'

'Now I'm in a job that I love more than anything I've done. So I think this has given me the opportunities to make those sorts of decisions, and it's been a really powerful experience.'

'Being able to revert back to old skills that could be reused in my new life.'

'Freedom to be able to drive again.'

'Achieving or doing hard things.'

'Doing things I was told that I wouldn't be able to do.'

'Stretching outside my comfort zone.'

'I feel that I have been so fortunate and I must help others who have not been so lucky to have recovered so well.'

'I am clearly meant to be in this world now and I have a responsibility to work…to be the best me I can possibly be.'

'I have a desire to share my story and feelings with others so they too can appreciate the wonders of life and all the moments they have…and let them know they're not alone.'

'I tell people I'm lucky to be alive, I'm lucky to have a family I've got — lucky now — if I'd had this 20 years ago I'd be locked away in an institution.'

'I felt so lucky that I'd survived.'

'I feel I am really lucky because this has happened to me, it has given me a chance to start my life again.'

'I feel special having experienced so many unique and valuable things.'

'I have to accept that I am newer better person and I have become more aware of the environment, pollution, good friendship, humanity to mankind, volunteering, service clubs and general sharing, better sailing skills (amazing eh).'

Some people I interviewed expressed how lucky they felt to have survived. Their experience had given them a chance to start their life again; they felt special because they had experienced so many unique and valuable things; they believed they are a newer, better person and had become more aware of things around them. Some had become highly sensitive to many things such as: noise, light, people, and even feelings. Brain injury had provided a really powerful learning experience for many of the participants.

Some people had come to realise that their brain injury had

provided some positive understanding. They had discovered that every day after the accident or medical emergency that nearly took their life was a bonus.

'It's like I'm constantly finding new aspects of myself.'

'I have a much greater understanding of life and people.'

I was astonished when several participants expressed the same thought — that after talking about their brain injury experience with the cage they now realised that their brain injury was both the worst and the best thing that had happened to them. Brain injury was the powerful experience that had led them to have epiphanies: to appreciate being alive, to be aware of their own strengths and weaknesses, to have a much greater understanding of life and people, to understanding what it was to feel older and in a lot of ways wiser. These people had the 'survivor's high'.

Hearing of these discoveries made me realise that this also has been my experience. Going through the challenge, putting in the great effort, struggling to grapple with and make sense of brain injury and life, has also led to me to appreciate being alive. I'm also aware of my strengths and weaknesses, and I feel a wiser person for the struggle. Getting the hang of living with brain injury has opened my eyes to the big picture of life.

> *'Actually it was a flower that told me one day that the world is really worth being in. It was a memorable experience because I was walking around the side of my house and the world had been grey for a long, long time and then I saw a red tulip, the bulb I'd put in a pot, and it had flowered red and honestly I stopped in my tracks, and it was like "wow", and I'll never forget that, and the world then had colour.'* (Irene)
>
> *'Yes, yes. I had a lightning bolt moment, an epiphany — in rehab I was in the ABI unit surrounded by others — you start comparing yourself and you say "I'm not as bad as them", and my family was saying "Oh my God, she isn't really quite with it!" and I knew I could sit back and do nothing, and let people look after me and pamper me for the rest of my life, or I could take*

another road and have a life that I felt I had achievement in. I felt I was at the crossroads that it was up to me — one was the hard slog the other was the easy road but I don't think I've ever taken the easy road.' (Jenny)

'I guess the secret to me, is to decide that this doesn't have to be permanent, that it doesn't have to be fully incapacitatory, and there's a lot I can do about it and to never give up…and to try anything and everything.' (Sarah)

'I'm glad this happened to me. My mother is horrified when I say that. But I would say that I haven't changed as a person, but I've learnt something… to be a little more courageous…I think this has given me the opportunities to make those sorts of decisions and it's been a really powerful experience and I'm glad it happened.' (Max)

As I've unlocked my brain I've discovered so many things about living and brain injury. I've realised that family and friends are priceless, manners are useful, acting can help me cope with others, a pat can be worth a thousand words, a good cry can be good, curiosity helps and knowing the story about how brain injury affects the whole person can help you know yourself.

Because of my sight and memory difficulties I had never read the published *Doing Up Buttons* and it was only in preparing for this new revised book that I finally understand the breadth of information I'd put together. When I wrote *Buttons* my brain was not sufficiently unlocked to remember or fully understand what I had written. Initially as I read the manuscript I became frustrated because I had spent four years doing a PhD, only to discover the truth of the information was in *Buttons* all along!

However, I now see that I have come a full circle. From being lost in the brain injury labyrinth I have travelled to the heart of the matter, and amazingly found happiness and a life worth living — things I thought were lost forever. It seems impossible that the damaged person I was, could, through thinking and unlocking my brain, acquire greater understanding of life, and be enriched by reflecting, searching, learning and gaining insight. Along with a huge number of people with brain injury I have proved that we must never, never, never, never, never, never, never ever give up hope!

Unlocking my brain has let me see that triumph is made up of two words — 'try' and 'umph', Together, with many other people with brain injury, I have found that we can do unattainable things we were told we would never be able to do. I have now discovered that impossible things can happen — pigs *can* fly!

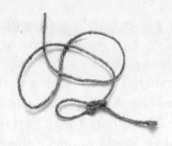

Further reading

Websites

In 1991, when I had my car accident and entered the labyrinth of acquired brain injury I had a great deal of trouble finding information. Today the reverse is true — there is a tsunami of information available at our fingertips on the internet.

People with brain injury and their families can search for information provided by brain injury support organisations such as:

AUSTRALIA
Brain Injury Australia: www.braininjuryaustralia.org.au
National Brain Injury Foundation: www.nbif.org.au
BrainLink: www.brainlink.org.au
Brain Injury Association of WA: www.headwest.asn.au
Brain Injury Association of NSW: www.biansw.org.au
Brain Injury Network of SA: www.binsa.org
NEW ZEALAND
The Brain Injury Association: www.brain-injury.org.nz
USA
Brain Injury Association of America: www.biausa.org

Brain Trauma Foundation: www.braintrauma.org
CANADA
Brain Injury Association of Canada: www.biac/aclc.ca (*Impact* weekly newsletter is excellent)
UNITED KINGDOM
Headway The Brain Injury Association: www.headway.org.uk

As well as brain injury support organisations it is possible to access studies and information published in academic journals, although these are often difficult to understand and interpret. The information in many websites uses unfamiliar language and ABI terminology as well as definitions that are 'problem-based' and biological.

As I reviewed many of the websites I had some difficulties — accessing information can be tricky for a person with memory, sight and other challenges. Many websites are busy with several columns, advertisements, colourful, moving images and other distracting material that makes it hard to find the required information. The layout of websites varies and when there are several bold headings it can be hard to work out where to start reading. Print size can also be a problem. Some websites have a 'font resize button' but this can be hard to find. It can also be difficult to revisit web based information when compared to reviewing material in a book. In books, important information can be highlighted for future reference and pages marked with paper or sticky notes.

On numerous occasions searching for information online about ABI has left me nauseated (due to my double vision — moving images, memory difficulties) and frustrated at the complexity the material. I assume many other people with ABI have had similar experiences.

If you Google *Traumatic Brain Injury Survival Guide* by Dr Glen Johnson, you will find easy-to-follow information presented in clear everyday language, with no distracting other material on the page. There are explanations, examples and advice presented in a friendly, positive and empathetic tone.

Many web pages isolate problems and classify them as physical, cognitive, behavioural and emotional, with smaller areas on social consequences and improvement, even though the effects of these problems overlap and influence each other. For example I Googled the following and found over a million results for each problem:

- **brain injury physical problems** (41,600,000 results). It is mind boggling to work out where to start looking at the information — balance, strength, co-ordination, sleep, vision, nausea, aphasia (difficulty articulating words), decreased smell or taste.
- **brain injury cognitive problems** (3,820,000 results). Information included thinking skills, trouble with attention and concentration, starting tasks, setting goals, memory, word finding, planning and organisation.
- **brain injury frustration and anger** (1,850,000 results). This search resulted in information about fear and anger about injuries, or problems that are caused by ABI anger, and how the anger threshold may be lowered.
- **brain injury emotional problems** (6,160,000 results). Information included mood swings, being on an emotional roller coaster, anxiety, nerves, fear, panic attacks, temper outbursts, irritability, depression, apathy, low self-esteem, uncontrollable emotional outbursts, agitation and unexplained anger, improper social communications, denial of changes, delusional paranoia, and excessive compulsive disorders.
- **brain injury post-traumatic stress disorder** (8,400,000 results). This search produced results including information on experiencing the trauma, fear that something bad will happen, physical symptoms and feeling detached.
- **brain injury severe depression** (2,920,000 results). Results included feeling 'low', 'down', and unhappy. People with

brain injury are several times more likely to develop major depression than the average person.
- **brain injury grief** (11,100,000 results). A majority of people with ABI experience loss and change resulting in grief.
- **brain injury behavioural problems** (20,300,000). This search produced information on personality changes, memory problems, difficulty with judgment, planning and problem solving, impulsive behaviour, and lack of initiative.
- **brain injury social consequences** (3,770,000 results). Brain injury indirectly contributes to the rising divorce, suicide, violent crimes, illicit drug and alcohol dependency and unemployment in society. People with brain injury are overrepresented in jails.

Do not despair! You are not alone!

Books written by people with ABI

In comparison to the style of information found on many websites, many of the books written by people with ABI have a more narrative and personal feel. These books often demonstrate a desire by people with ABI to tell their story and to remind readers about hope and determination, to let people know that life can be good, despite changed identity and circumstances. The stories explain 'I am not who you see', 'I am really a combination of who "I was" and who "I am"'. They want to tell the story of how the calamity happened — the fall, the car accident, the stroke, the mugging or the black ice. The books are generally written in an easy-to-read style using everyday words to express the struggle, the complexities and the difficulties of ABI. They reiterate again and again that understanding and knowledge is power to the brain damaged person, and that people with ABI and their families should never give up.

Some books depict the day-to-day frustrations of living with brain injury like Osborn's *Over my head: A Doctor's Own Story of Head Injury from the Inside Looking Out* (1997). She leads us to contrast her pre-brain-injury life as a medical doctor, with her post brain-injury-life where she has difficulty showering and dressing. Nine years post-injury she believes that she is still improving due to learnt strategies. Not only does she tell about what it is like to have ABI, she gives hope as we read of her progress from confusion, grief, loss, dysfunction and alienation to a happy life.

Some books focus on the loss of identity. Becker (2004), author of a *New York Times* bestseller, tackles the big issue of ABI — identity: what makes us us in *I had brain surgery, what's your excuse?*

A thread that runs through some stories is the importance of acceptance. Skloot, author of 17 books, novelist, poet and essayist, wrote his book to tell how he came to accept his injury in *In the Shadow of Memory* (2003).

Some books focus on how the person is treated by other people. Calderwood's *Cracked: Recovering after brain injury* (2003) tells of her struggle to discover her identity and come to terms with her disability and the sense of loss, grief and rage that it had taken nine months to be diagnosed. Mason's (2009) book *Head cases: Stories of brain injury and its aftermath* narrates her struggle to return to independent living from a vegetative state after being hit by a drunk driver while cycling.

Garrison's *Don't leave me this way: or when I get back on my feet you'll be sorry* (2007) tells us how she woke up in hospital after a substantial stroke and thought that she had survived for a reason or a purpose.

Another issue written about by people with ABI is their rehabilitation experience. Strand, *Meditations on Brain Injury* (2004), writes about how the controlled and structured environment of rehabilitation reminded him of elementary school. Because he was not informed of the reason for doing certain tasks, he believed he was expected to agree to complete the task and he resumed the outlook and behaviour he'd had when he was at school. He didn't realise he was completing tasks to benefit himself, rather he thought it was his duty to please the rehabilitation professional, which resulted in his learning very little. He now realises that if he'd understood the reason for completing tasks he would have been more engaged in his learning experience.

Sherry's doctoral thesis, published as *If only I had a brain: Deconstructing brain injury* (2006), focuses on the need for a new way to understand and react to the brain injury experience. It talks about the person with brain injury's rights, including the right to make choices and have respect.

Meili's *Going the Distance* (2003), written 14 years after she was assaulted and raped as she jogged in Central Park, New York, identifies many of the reasons why people with ABI write books. She was looking for a way to turn what was truly horrible into something positive; the attack, meant to take her life, instead gave her life greater meaning. She writes about the capacity of the human body and the human spirit to heal and the power of the mind. She believes that the heart is as important as medicine in healing, and even though she still suffers from her injuries her experience has let her find her own humanity, kindness and love.

Many of these books tell of the importance of love, faith, acceptance, gratitude, humility, compassion, hope and beauty.

Books written by people with ABI with their family members

Some books are written by family members of people with brain injury. These include Bob and Lee Woodruff's (2008) book *In an instant: A family's journey of love and healing*. This tells of Bob Woodruff's experience after he was injured by a roadside bomb while an anchor of *ABC News* in Iraq. Bob and Lee Woodruff have since established the Bob Woodruff Foundation to raise money to provide resources to the estimated 320,000 service members who have sustained traumatic brain injury (TBI) and estimated 300,000 service members who have probable psychological wounds.

Some books aim to help the person with ABI to obtain power, by helping them to understand their injury. Jameson and Jameson's *Brain injury survivor's guide: Welcome to our world* (2007) contains advice to others with brain injury and they assert that for the brain injured person knowledge is power. Kelley's *My Brain Gets Full* (2010) describes the effects of brain injury, his denial and the deficits that will not go away, techniques that help him manage and his legal battle for compensation. Brennan, (2002), a professor of English with special interest in memory, 'jump-started' the memory of her daughter who had ABI by constantly retelling her story and fostering creativity and humour (traits she had before her brain injury). She states that the book *Being with Rachel, a personal story of memory and survival* was a combined endeavour.

Books written by family members

A number of books have been written by family members of people with ABI (Biagioni, 2004; Brennan, 2002; Camp, 2005; Coenig, 2008; Cohen, 2003; Crimmins, 2000; Cromer, 2006; Johansen, 2002; Johns, 2005; Lash, 1993; Morningstar, 1998; Rocchio, 2004). These can be found through a Google search using the person's name plus the words 'brain injury'.

Several people have written accounts telling of the experience of a family adapting to life with a brain injured person, giving hope and motivation to others with ABI and raising awareness of ABI. Themes include grief, loss, love, hope, acceptance and adaptation.

For example Thomas's (2006) book *A three dog life: A memoir* about her husband who sustained ABI was selected as one of the best books of 2006 by the *LA Times* and the *Washington Post*. The book demonstrates how tragedy can bend, but not break some relationships. Thomas writes of grief and guilt as she shows that a new life can be built upon tragedy.

Stories published on the internet

ABI support organisations now publish the stories of people with ABI. Googling 'brain injury stories' identifies some 37,300,000 results — Survivor Stories, Personal Stories, Brain Injury Stories, Your Stories Brain Injury Australia, Headway My Story, Brain Injury Stories: Brain Injury online, and Living with TBI: Personal Stories to name just a few.

Stories written by people with ABI appear to have a common theme of never giving up, the importance of hope and trying to express what it is like to live a changed life, as well as recognition that self-help can be an important part of the process of adaptation and coping.

Charles H Perkhurst said that 'purpose gives life meaning'. As people with brain injury and family members of people with brain injury we are presented with a strong purpose — to try to capture a worthwhile life. In looking for a purpose 'The most important thing about getting somewhere is starting right where you are.' (Bruce Fairchild Barton)

Theodore Roosevelt said 'Do what you can, with what you have, where you are.' My purpose has been to find 'string', a step by step journey into the labyrinth of brain injury to discover helpful information. Now that I have found a trail, I can make my way out into the light.

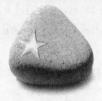

Index

acceptance 52, 95–6, 187–9
    new self, of 118–19, 173
achievement, sense of 112–13, 119
acquired brain injury (ABI) 12–13, 24, 190–1
    advice 141
    bodily temperature control 84
    communication problems 23, 33, 34–5, 39, 50, 74–5, 126, 140, 141, 177
    complexity 171
    effects 41
    help and support, need for 43
    images for understanding 150–2
    insight, acquiring 156–68
    Keys to the ABI Cage *see* Keys to the ABI Cage
    lack of explanations 41, 43, 59, 61–2, 125–6
    learning theories 170
    learning to understand 186
    motor ability and control 41
    perceptions, misleading 42
    personal stories of 57–8, 60, 153–5, 166–7
    power of experience 189–90
    presentations on experience of 150–2
    reactions from people 102–3, 174
    sensations 20–1, 26–7, 40

strategies 127, 186
support organisations 165
understanding of ramifications 126–7, 140–1, 186
activities, difficulties with 49–50, 66, 105
aggression 43
anger 70, 94, 170, 178
animals 36–7, 39, 72
appetite, poor 32, 40, 175
Azar, Dr 139

balance 34, 40, 41, 50, 59, 79, 115, 176, 179
group balance classes 56, 60
behaviour
extremes 114
inappropriate 90, 179
birds 91–2, 134–7
fantail doves 135–7, 163
bitterness 46–7, 107
blaming self 67–8
blood clots 32
bone specialist 97, 98
boredom 66, 108
brachial plexus injury 24
brain scans 28, 58

catheter 31
challenges, coping with 150–2
chest infections 87, 115
choking 25, 32, 37
claustrophobia 94
clavicle injury 24, 29, 36
closed head injury 23
clumsiness 33, 37, 65
commonsense and judgment 90
communication 23, 33, 34–5, 39, 74–5, 90, 126, 141, 177
comprehension 90
concentration 42, 48, 50, 56, 81, 89
confidence 59
loss of 173
confusion 23, 33, 40–1, 44, 62, 89, 153–4, 176
coordination 41, 50
'Coping Cake' 151–2

coping mechanisms 120-1, 150-2
court cases
    assessment for 96-9
    civil action 96-102
    Criminal Court 93-6, 99
creative side of brain 120
Criminal Court 93-6, 99
crisis intervention 43

de Horne, David 100
dependence 33, 42, 44, 51, 75-6, 104-5
depersonalisation 42
depression 31, 43, 44, 170, 178
depth perception 41, 50
determination 132-3
diplopia 23
Disability Liaison Officers 157
disorientation 42-3, 115, 121
dizziness 135
Doing Up Buttons 12, 13, 152-3, 163, 190
dreams 27, 34-5, 43

eating difficulties 32-3, 37, 75
emotional control 90, 170
emotional problems 177-8
emotional support 43
empathy, need for 124-5, 174
employment, return to 63, 77-85
    longing for 78-9, 107
    support 59, 78
encouragement, need for 61, 131
epilepsy 20, 34-5, 61, 86-8
    reaction to medication 87-8
exhaustion 56, 100, 101, 135, 176-7
eye injury 24, 85
eye patches 28, 38, 53, 64-5, 82, 84-5, 113
eye surgeon 65, 99
eye tests 98
eyesight *see* vision

facial expressions, reading 41
fairness 173

families 174
    celebrations 115–16
    parents 128–33
    responses from 27–8, 43, 50, 51–2, 65–6, 71, 115, 124–5, 135
    responses to 25–6, 39, 91–2, 124–5
    role reversals 75–6
fate 169–70
fatigue 77, 157 *see also* exhaustion; tiredness
faulty thinking 67
fear 29, 43, 44, 58
Fedor, Deborah 141–2
5th Congress on Brain Injury 153
finances 101–2
floating sensation 20, 40, 56, 65, 79
friends 104, 174
    responses from 42
    responses to 26, 42
frustration 43, 44, 64, 70, 90, 105, 117–18, 154, 178
    dealing with 119

goals 106, 108–9, 112
'golden spoons' 151–2
Gordon, Dr 142–3
GP 49, 55, 61, 99, 118
gratitude 45–7
grief 61–2, 119, 141, 169
guilt 25, 37, 41, 43, 67–8, 103, 154, 170, 174, 179

happiness 70
hatred 46–7, 61
Head Injury Association, Brooklyn 139–40
Head Injury Service 152
Headway Victoria 41, 42
health professionals 28, 33, 49, 55–6, 64–5, 84–5, 86, 99, 113, 125–6
    judgmentalism 59–60, 97, 173
    opinions on 180–1
    tests 28, 56, 59, 96–9, 100
helping someone else 108–9
home, returning to 36–44
hope 12, 110–11, 168
Hope Stones 152, 153
hopelessness 58

hospital 31–5, 42, 70, 124
    general ward 21, 23–30
    intensive care unit 19–22
    procedures 27–9, 31
    rehabilitation 57–62
    tests 28–9
humiliation 28

independence, loss of 33
Independent Living Center 142
information 192–199
    books 195–199
    need for 43, 138–44, 153, 186
    websites 192–5
insanity, feelings of 29, 35, 41, 44, 179
intensive care unit 19–22
International Philosophy for Children 16
internet
    search terms 194–5
    stories published on 199
IQ tests 97
irrationality 43
isolation 41, 49, 108, 179
Ivanhoe Girls' Grammar 17, 93

Keller, Helen 131
Keys to the ABI Cage 163, 164
    active learning 170
    analysis 169–71
    creation of 165
    interviews 166–7
    participants 165–6, 171
    'sad', 'mad' and 'bad' 178–9
    talk-about cards 165, 178
    themes 163, 164
knowledge, gaining 109

learning theories 170
light sensitivity 25
loneliness 108
loss 61–2, 169, 172–3

Malloy, Dr Maureen 125–6
marriage 70–2, 124–5, 141
medical bills 99
medication 87
  epilepsy, for 87–8
  painkillers 37
  reaction to 87–8
memory 40, 79, 82–3, 119, 126, 127
  long-term 41
  short-term 41, 42
Mt Sinai Hospital 142–3
music 26–7, 48, 50, 66, 107, 143

nausea 40
neurologist 55–6, 64–5, 86, 99
New York 138–44
nightmares 27
noise, sensitivity to 23, 25, 26, 29, 42, 43, 48–9, 109
'normality' 175–6

occupational therapy 56, 60
'old' and 'new' selves 173
one-sided neglect of brain 42, 64
optician 113
optimism 110–11
osteopath 99, 135
outings 53, 69–72
overreactions 43, 67
oxygen 27, 31, 34

pain 20–2, 23, 24, 27, 28–9, 31, 33, 34, 37–9, 43, 44, 56, 58, 66, 94–5
painkillers 31, 33–4, 37–8
panic 29, 37, 94, 115
  attacks 50, 119
parents 128–33, 154
peace and quiet 109 *see also* noise, sensitivity to
personality changes 66–7
pessimism 110–11
philosophy 16
  enrichment sessions 80, 81–4, 134
  Master's degree 16, 17, 73–6
physical injuries 20, 23–4, 36

        long-lasting effects 106
physiotherapists 28, 31, 49, 56, 59–60, 65, 76, 99
pleasure 118
        lack of 66–7, 108, 118
pneumonia 20, 24, 32
pneumothorax 24, 27
poetry 112–13
post-traumatic amnesia 23
post-traumatic stress disorder 42–3, 62
powerlessness 96, 178
progress 187–8
        measuring 75
psychiatrists 97–8
psychological support 43, 118–22, 123–4
psychologist 56, 56, 97–8

Ramcharan, Dr Paul 157
reading 27, 50, 49, 74–5, 117
reality and unreality 34–5, 86–8
recovery 113, 115
        coping 113
        lack of 61, 63
        time for 61
redefinition of self 119
rehabilitation 34, 42, 55–62, 142, 171, 179–81
        group balance classes 56, 60
        lack of explanations 59–60, 61–2
        report 79–80
        tests 59
religious beliefs 175
resources 192–199
        books written by family members 198–199
        books written by people with ABI 195–8
        websites 192–5
ribs, injury to 20, 23–4, 36, 106–7
routine, development of 108–9
Ryder, Dr John 140

self-help 142
senses, impaired 41
shame 28, 170, 174–5
shopping 49, 50, 53, 61–2, 75, 79

short-term memory 41, 42
simplicity 109
sleeping problems 176-7
smell, sense of 32, 40, 41, 48, 50, 65
'snakes' and 'ladders' 151
social contact, withdrawal from 90, 114
spasms 38
spatial problems 41
speaking difficulties 74-5, 79
speech therapy 56, 59
stiffness 39
stigma 174-5
stress relief 109-10
studying 73-6
    PhD on brain injury 157-8
swallowing difficulties 21, 25

'Talk About Change' 13, 150-5, 157
Taste 32, 40, 41, 48, 50
teaching 15-17, 54, 77-85, 107
    philosophy and discussion sessions 80, 81-4, 134
thinking and attitude 149
time
    concept of 56-7, 63-4, 78
    limits on recovery period 61, 181
    structuring 108
tiredness 69, 77, 84, 108, 121
tongue injury 20, 21
touch, sense of 65
travel 114-15
trust 169
    loss of 175
    'new self', of 173
    others, of 174
tubes 34

unhappiness 66-7, 105, 117-18, 154

vision 20, 41, 48, 49, 64, 79, 90, 176
    double 27, 38, 40, 42, 64-5, 77, 80, 139, 176
    interpretation of information 41, 114
    painted contact lens 113-14

              'scanning' 59, 79
              tests 28
visuo-spatial ability 90

walking 50, 65, 79, 89, 94
              stick, using 59, 82
warmth 49, 118
websites 192–5
weeping 50–1, 66, 70, 80–1, 85
whiplash injury 24
workaholic, being 108
Workcare and Transport Accident Commission 96, 97, 153
worthlessness, feelings of 37, 42, 71, 170
              tackling 119–20
writing 105, 112–13
              difficulties with 82